Intermittent Fasting for Women

Joy Cooper

Table of Contents

Introduction

Fasting? Can I do it?

Am I capable of fasting?

How long should I fast?

What's the point of fasting?

Is it healthy?

Will I lose weight fast?

These and many more questions arise when we talk about Intermittent Fasting. When the word fasting is mentioned, we often think of hunger pangs, people with no energy, and walking around looking pale. Fasting is often associated with unpleasant physical reactions.

And with all of the misconceptions out there about fasting, it is hard to see how this could be healthy. This book is going to take some time to discuss intermittent fasting a bit more, and why it is such a great eating plan to help you reach your goals.

In addition to talking about the different parts of intermittent fasting, we will also spend some time talking about other important aspects including exercising, staying motivated, and making sure that you get the most out of this eating plan. So what about intermittent fasting then? Is it harder than the normal fast?

To plenty of people, intermittent fasting is one of the easiest forms of diet to lose weight (well yes, if you are fasting, the idea is to lose weight), but intermittent fasting has more benefits than just losing weight. For some people, fasting intermittently is a healthier way to lose weight compared to restrictive diets.

For some, it's about giving the digestive system a break, and for some, it is a great way to maintain a healthy glucose balance. In this book, we will explore intermittent fasting as a healthy way for weight loss and also a pathway towards a healthier way of living.

Before we begin, there is one thing that you should note when it comes to intermittent fasting – it is *not* going to work the same way for both men and women. Why? For one very simple reason – men and women's bodies are simply made to function differently. Intermittent fasting, just like every other form of diet method on the market, is not going to be as simple as having one solution that fixes everyone's problems.

To fully reap the benefits of intermittent fasting, you are going to need to do what works best for your body. Everyone has got a different type of body, and you are going to need to learn to *listen to your body* to see maximum results.

By the end of this book, you are going to know everything that you need to make an informed decision about intermittent fasting specifically catered to women. When you begin, you are going to start off on the right foot because, at the end of the day, it is all about getting the desired results you want to see.

As with any diet or new lifestyle change, be sure to consult your doctor before you get started to make sure that it is a safe option for you. When you are ready, your journey towards better health is about to begin right now.

Should I go on an Intermittent Fast?

That depends - what are your body or weight goals? According to Carly Pollack, a Certified Clinical Nutritionist as well as a Lifestyle Coach at Nutritional Wisdom, says that our body is designed to burn energy by using glucose or fat. When you make your body become adapted to fat as fuel, it will start using fat for energy instead of carbohydrates broken to glucose.

When you intermittent fast, you create a superior environment for your body to burn fat. Of course, there are other benefits to intermittent fasting which we will look into in this book. This involves cancer prevention, longevity, improved digestion as well as insulin resistance. So the bottom line is, doing intermittent fasting is a personal choice based on what your health goals are.

You can go on an intermittent fast to kick start a more superior process of your digestive system, lose weight healthily, and also reap the benefits of having better insulin tolerance.

Who should not try intermittent fasting?

Just like other diets and eating plants, intermittent fasting is also not for everyone. There are medical conditions that prevent people from taking on intermittent fasting. The main issues are:

- People with a history of eating disorders
- People who are currently underweight
- People are recovering from illness or injury
- People who have Type 1 diabetes mellitus
- People with low blood pressure (hypotension)
- Women who are trying to conceive
- Women who are pregnant

The reason why those in the group above are listed is that while there are positive benefits, there could be risks of impairment, risk of dangerously low sugar levels, or even the risk of not getting enough nutrition. Now that you have an idea of who can and who cannot go on intermittent fasting, let's have a look at a few basic things regarding this fast.

Women, especially women who are suffering from hormonal imbalances, adrenal dysfunction, any other sort of bodily imbalance, and even those who suffer from thyroid problems should be very wary about starting an intermittent fasting plan. You can consult your doctor beforehand and just consult with them if this is going to be a safe bet for you or not, but if you are thinking about starting this eating regime, you should be cautious as it may cause your body more harm than good. Women with PCOS, for example, could experience problems with intermittent fasting because it will begin to take its toll on your body and regular fasting may be in danger of causing your body more stress instead of helping it get healthier. Among some of the problems that women with hormonal imbalances could encounter if they undergo the intermittent fasting program includes acne, depression, stress, and even disruptions in your menstrual cycle. The bottom line is that women with any kind of hormonal imbalances *should not* be doing intermittent fasting because your body is already not functioning the way that a healthy body should, and fasting is only going to increase the severity of the imbalances you are already experiencing.

Intermittent fasting is great, that is unless you have adrenal, thyroid, or autoimmune issues. Although intermittent fasting is supposed to be the way to get your health back on track again, it isn't going to work as well for those who are already not in the peak of health because you're most likely already struggling. Pregnant women should stay well away from intermittent fasting too because you are at a stage where your body *needs* to have all the nutrients it can get to feed the growing baby inside of you. Weight gain is to be expected during pregnancy. That is just something that you have to deal with, it's a packaged deal.

The Three Rules of Intermittent Fasting

- Drink water when you are thirsty. When you are fasting, continue doing this without fail.
- You can also exercise while fasting- we will explore this even more in the book. It is totally safe as long as you do not overexert yourself.
- Consult your doctor before you go on fasts and also if any medications can be consumed when you are fasting.

Chapter 1- What is Intermittent Fasting?

Intermittent fasting is a simple yet very powerful concept of alternating feasting and fasting patterns.

When you intermittent fast, you change your eating patterns of fasting and eating periods. It is not about eliminating a food group or increasing the intake of a specific food group and reducing the number of other food groups. In fact, it has nothing to do with the foods you eat. It's about WHEN you should be eating.

It can solve the highly complex problem of obesity and fat loss through simple measures. However, weight loss is only one of the smaller benefits of intermittent fasting. There are more benefits to intermittent fasting than just weight loss such as eliminating or reducing chronic and complex health issues like diabetes, cardiovascular disorders, chronic inflammation, etc.

This may look like a tall claim, but all the facts are backed by various scientific studies carried out all over the globe. Its practical applications and ease of use have made intermittent fasting such a craze.

There are different ways to fast intermittently whether by a week or by day which we will definitely cover in this book. Intermittent fasting can seem like a fad, much like how all other diets have become fads. People worry that fasting is going to be unhealthy for them. They worry that it is going to be too hard.

But Why Fast?

Although it is a method which has been around for a long time practiced through religion and culture, it is only in recent years that intermittent fasting has gained traction to become currently one of the most popular fitness and health trends in the world. Yes, this ancient secret of changing your eating ways to develop a healthier lifestyle is no longer a secret. But wait, *why* is it referred to as the ancient secret to humans achieving better health?

It is ancient because, as mentioned earlier, this technique and precise way of eating has been around for a long time, and something which – believe it or not – has been practiced and recorded throughout human history for as long as we can remember.

This ancient secret has been around for so long that it is – in fact – ancient. It is just that before this, we may not have paid much attention to it. You've probably already experienced several times throughout your life when you intermittent fasted, only that you were not aware that you were doing so.

This ancient secret habit was almost forgotten, but now, the benefits that it brings has thrust this diet into the spotlight. With the current lifestyle that many of us are living, the pursuit for better health is one that many are rushing towards.

Believe it, intermittent fasting is a method that has been around since, quite possibly, when the earliest humans were around. It's true. Think about it, early humans needed to hunt and gather their food. They couldn't just walk into the supermarket and pick out what they needed, not the way we do today.

Back then, if you wanted to eat, you needed to hunt, and there was no option of keeping the food they gained that day in the refrigerator either, where it would be conveniently available to them anytime that they wanted.

Since hunting was so unpredictable, there would be times when they would have had to go without food if there was nothing to be caught that day. This lifestyle was responsible for helping them condition their bodies to effectively function even in the absence of food for an extended period of time.

Thus, intermittent fasting was born. Fasting is something that is much more natural to the human body than eating small meals several times a day. That is because our bodies, since the days of the early humans, have been accustomed to it. They survived on it.

Since then, man has continually progressed and move forward, and intermittent fasting was no longer just a means of survival. This method too evolved with the times, and now fasting is done for several reasons. One example would be for either spiritual or religious purposes. Some of the world's major religions, including Buddhism, Islam, Judaism, and Christianity commonly practice fasting.

Intermittent fasting is not exactly a diet, but rather, it is an eating plan. With this plan, you would be regulating the periods of when you would be eating and when you would be fasting. Instead of randomly and haphazardly missing your meals like you may have done in the past, this time you would be mindfully and purposefully scheduling your meals to precise eating intervals to reap the maximum benefits from this method.

Intermittent fasting is quite possibly one of the easiest and simplest techniques out there for you to take off the weight, and more importantly, keep it off for good. The secret behind its effectiveness is because it is going to require very little change on your part. The change portion of the weight loss process is where most diets and people tend to fail, because often that change doesn't bring them any happiness or is too difficult to pursue for a long time. That is why it becomes so easy to fall back into old patterns and eating habits.

Why intermittent fasting is so beneficial is because it isn't just another crazy diet fad that is going to put your body through extreme periods only to crash and burn later. It isn't just another fad that holds empty promises of losing weight fast only to gain it all back again because the diet was too stressful to keep up with. It is a *way of eating* that is going to get you leaner, fitter, and healthier without all the craziness of drastically cutting down your calories or severely depriving yourself of food. Intermittent fasting is all about *you*.

The great thing about intermittent fasting is that you do not feel as though you are being forced to do anything you don't want to. In fact, this is probably the only weight loss eating plan where you will be in full control of the choices that you may. You choose when you want to begin your fast.

You choose when you want to end your fast. You can start your fast, and you can stop your fast if you feel the need to. If you don't feel like you are up for a round of intermittent fasting today, that's okay because there is always tomorrow. This is the only "diet" plan where you have the power to control the outcome.

With intermittent fasting, what you are going to be doing is not eating for a certain window period. This window time frames are broken down into two categories, which are the 16-hour fasting periods and the 24-hour fasting periods. If you are going with the 24-hour option, you are only going to need to do this two times a week, because depriving yourself of food for too long will only send your body into fat conservation mode, which is what you want to avoid.

What benefits should a balanced and healthy body bring me?

A healthy individual is one who also has a clean bill of health. If you haven't had a regular or recent check-up with your local GP, you should get one before you begin the intermittent fasting method. An individual with a clean bill of health is at a lower risk of contracting any deadly diseases which include cardiovascular problems, diabetes, arthritis, and more. This is what you should strive to be.

Exercising regularly is something that you need to start doing if you're not already doing it. If you want to be healthy, exercise is going to have to be a part of that package. Not only does it help to regulate your body's blood flow, but it also helps to balance out and boost your metabolism, which goes without saying is needed for overall good health.

When you are in good health, here is what's going to happen:

- **You Become a More Confident Person** – Living a healthy lifestyle can do wonders for your mental and emotional health. You're going to start feeling really good about yourself because you like the results that you see in the mirror. A healthy diet and regular exercise will give your body that healthy look and glow that no cosmetic product or makeup would ever replicate because that glow is going to come from within. When you know that you look good, you start to feel good. You're energetic, you're clear-minded, you feel good, and you feel like you are ready to take on any challenge that is thrust at you. You become a more confident person.

- **You're Emotionally More Stable** – Our emotional state is linked to good health because believe it or not, the mood is psychosomatic. When your body does not feel good, don't expect your mind to be feeling all that great either. Mood swings will become inevitable when a person experiences hormonal ups and downs as a result of poor health. If you find this hard to believe, just think of a time when you came down with a cold and felt fantastic emotionally. Almost certainly the answer is going to be *never* because it is impossible for us to feel any kind of happy when our bodies are not working as it should be. That is a perfect example of why good health is so important because being healthy will help your body boost its serotonin levels, which is also known as the happiness hormone. Yes, that hormone exists, why do you think you get that rush of happiness when you consume alcohol or ice cream for example? Because of the temporary spike in serotonin that you just received. What to feel that way all the time? Be healthy.

- **You Obviously Look Much Better** – This goes without saying. Sugary drinks, fatty foods, and junk food may give you a temporary glow and feeling of happiness, but that is only going to be short-lived. Why? Because eating too much junk like that is also going to cause you wrinkles and some extra, unwanted padding around your waist. Plus, it makes you feel lethargic and sluggish when you are carrying around more weight than you should, which is what a lot of obese people feel like all the time. Being healthy and consuming enough water, getting ample sleep, and eating a nutritious diet packed with fruits, vegetables, grains, protein, and more is the secret to keeping your skin looking healthy and your hair shiny. Not only are you going to find that you look better, but your movements are going to become a lot more energized, which will give you an overall look for appearing more attractive, youthful, and supple.

- **You Become More Productive** – Because we can't always rely on coffee and tobacco to give us that spike in energy that we need. It's only a momentary spike and it won't last long, wouldn't you prefer having that feeling all day long? A balanced lifestyle and good health are how you achieve that same spike in energy that coffee can give you each morning. Cut down that dependency of getting your energy sources from elsewhere and instead, just choose good health to feel that way all the time.

Chapter 2 - Understanding Weight, Obesity, and Its Impact on Women

In the United States, more than 2 in 3 women are obese or overweight. The fact that you're overweight also means that it has a high probability of leading to plenty of diseases that affect women (and also men) such as diabetes, heart diseases as well as certain types of cancer. Talking about your weight can be uncomfortable to plenty of people but if you find a medical practitioner such as a doctor or a nurse that you are comfortable with, they can be a valuable partner in your journey to lose weight.

How would you know if you are obese or overweight?

Apart from the physical aspects which are the most obvious signs, another good indicator is to look at our Body Mass Index (BMI). This index can be used to determine if your weight is in a healthy range with your height. This tool helps to estimate your body fat and you use your height x weight into the BMI calculator created by the Centers for Disease Control and Prevention.

This BMI indicator just gives you an indication of how healthy your weight is. However, this does not, by any means, count as accurate. The BMI count is less accurate for some people compared to others. For instance, for people who are muscular, their BMI may be above 25 because muscle weighs more than fat.

Another good way to understand the healthiness of your weight is by looking at your waist circumference. Weight researchers and doctors agree that women with a circumference of their waist larger than 35 inches are considered overweight or obese.

What is the cause of obesity?

A person becomes obese when their body ends up storing more calories than it uses. Your body does need calories such as minerals, essential vitamins, and nutrients for it to remain healthy and active. If your body uses less of these calories than it stores, this will cause you to gain weight.

Other causes can also be a person's environment over a lifetime that can cause obesity. This is in relation to the food you eat but it could also be influenced by other factors that are not within your control such as availability of healthy food, pollution, or even access to safe places to exercise such as gyms or even parks.

How common are obesity and overweight?

At least where the United States is concerned, it is very common. Women of all races, ages, and ethnicities can be obese and overweight. However, in some groups, overweight and obesity are more prevalent. Apart from food and external factors, there are other factors that cause obesity which are things like family background, past events, and the place where you live.

If you find it hard to exercise or incorporate any kind of physical activity or you are worried about your weight, you can speak to a doctor or dietician. Also, there could be some risk factors that cause obesity and overweight that are beyond your control. Your dietician, doctor, or nurse would be able to recommend healthier eating habits as well as exercises to help you reach a more optimal weight.

Also, there could be some medication that could cause weight gain so this is something you need to tell your doctor if you are in the process of changing the way you eat and live.

What individual factors unique to me can make it more likely that I'll gain weight?

Obesity affects a person in many different ways and this can happen over a long period of time. The factors that influence our weight are:

- Our family background and genes - There is not just one 'fat' gene. Obesity runs in families and there are different genes that work to make a person more likely to gain weight. The situation that you are in also affects your genes and this could have begun at infancy based on the eating and physical activity instilled in you by your parents or caregiver when you were a child.

- Your Metabolism - Some people are blessed with very good metabolism. Metabolism is the ability of your body to burn calories and this affects your weight gain or weight loss. Men who are muscular, for instance, burn more calories quickly. Women's metabolism might change throughout their lives depending on changes that take place during puberty, pregnancy as well as menopause.

- Your age - Of course, your metabolism gets slower the older you get. We also tend to lose muscle as we age and the less muscle means we burn calories less.

- Any trauma - The traumatic events that have taken place in our lives are something that we may not have control over and this can cause either weight gain or weight loss. Women (and yes, men too) who experience negative events during childhood, such as abuse, parental divorce, or road accidents can lead to obesity in adults. Girls who are sexually abused, research has pointed out, are more likely to gain weight when they become adults and eventually lead to obesity. Those that experience PTSD also are highly likely to gain weight as well.

- Medication could also lead to weight gain. Medicines related to sleep and mental health can lead to weight gain or it could also make it difficult to lose weight. If you are taking any prescriptions that may cause you to put on weight or make it difficult to lose weight, you should let your doctor know about it.

- Not getting enough sleep can also cause weight gain simply because it affects your hormone levels and that affects your food choices as well as your appetite. Not being well-rested also affects whether you have the energy for exercise throughout the day.

How can the location of where I live make it more likely that I'll gain weight?

The surroundings in which we live in may be a cause of weight gain in people. These things are such as:

- **Your neighborhood** - Look around you and see how safe or easy it is for you to exercise? There are some neighborhoods that do not have parks or sidewalks or even a gym nearby that makes it difficult to do even simple physical activities such as brisk walking or running. There could be traffic or even safety issues with even taking your dog out for a walk. Some places can also be unsafe for those with disabilities too.

- **Your access to healthy food** - Our access to healthy food also influences our weight gain. Healthy food can be expensive and many people do not have the luxury of low-cost healthy options for food at the places where they live. It could also be that your route to and from work or school has the most fast-food restaurants than access to a grocery store where you can get fresh produce.

- **Pollution in your area** - Things like secondhand smoke and air pollution (like haze) is also linked to obesity. Chemicals also exist in the food we eat so if there's pollution, there is also a likelihood that it has permeated into your food too and this leads to obesity.

What are the effects on women who are overweight?

Obesity has indirectly led to millions of deaths each year in America. It's been said over and over again that being overweight and/or obese increases the risks of serious health issues.

Let's just go over the basic complications:

- **You would have breathing problems** - Sleep apnea is a common occurrence for women who are obese or overweight. Sleep apnea makes you stop breathing for a while or your breathing becomes shallow while you sleep and this is due to the fat in the neck which narrows the airflow. Those with sleep apnea do not get enough oxygen to their brain while sleeping and this will eventually lead to heart diseases.

- **You increase your risk of different types of cancer** - Your cancer risks increase tenfold if you are overweight or obese, bringing up your risk factor to a total of 13 different kinds of cancer from endometrial, rectal, stomach, gallbladder, esophagus, kidney, liver, multiple myeloma as well as ovarian and thyroid cancer.

- **You also become diabetic -** As a person who is obese or overweight, the likelihood of you getting diabetes is twice as high. Eating right and exercise can prevent this from happening as the right foods and burning calories helps control our blood sugar levels.

- **You increase your risk of Heart disease -** The more you weigh, the higher your risk of heart disease. That's a given. For women, this is a leading cause of death, apart from breast cancer, in the United States. Even if your family has no history of heart diseases, this risk becomes more prevalent if you are obese.

- **High blood pressure & high cholesterol -** Getting high blood pressure is common among people who are overweight and obese. Of course, losing weight reduces this risk. High blood pressure affects your arteries, damaging it and this will cause more problems such as heart diseases and stroke. This would also lead to excess fat in your body. Obesity increases LDL cholesterol, which is the bad one and lowers the HDL which is the good cholesterol. When this happens, bad cholesterol increases a buildup of fatty plaque in the arteries. When we start exercising, this fatty plaque starts to burn off and helps keep our HDL and LDL at healthy levels.

- **There might be pregnancy problems** - There could be problems that arise during pregnancy if you are obese or overweight. These complications could be things like gestational diabetes or dangerously high blood pressure. There is a more serious condition that occurs when you're obese which is called preeclampsia. Getting regular and early prenatal care will help you lessen or prevent necessary risks and lead to a healthy pregnancy. Of course, losing weight and exercising will also lead to a healthier pregnancy.

- **Your risk of Stroke increases** - When we carry extra body fat around our waist, the risk of stroke increases.

Lowering your weight to even 3% to 5% can reduce a multitude of health risks. If you weigh 160 pounds, losing between 5 and 8 pounds itself can make you healthier.

Does it matter where on my body I carry the weight?

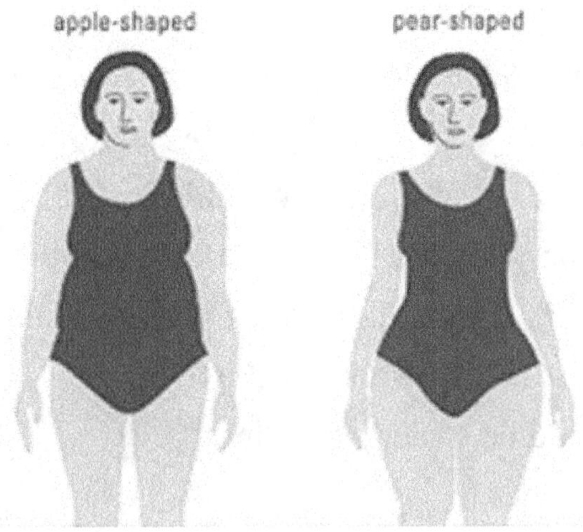

Where you carry your weight matters and it makes a huge difference in your health. Belly fat is much more dangerous compared to fat in different areas of the body.

Women with apple-shaped and pear-shaped body types

Women who are apple-shaped tend to carry more fat in the belly area while those who are pear-shaped have more fat in their hips and thighs. Extra weight is never healthy however, women who are apple-shaped are at a higher risk for certain health risks such as type 2 diabetes, heart diseases as well as colorectal cancer. The reason for this is that the type of fat your body stores in the abdomen is a different kind of fat compared to the ones in your hips and thighs.

While the BMI count does tell us how much fat we have in our body, it does not tell us where our weight is concentrated more. You need to measure your waist size by standing up straight and using a tape measure around your middle, just right above the hip bones. Your ideal waist size should be less than half of your height. If you are 6 feet tall, your waist size should be less than 36 inches whereas, if you are 5 feet 4 inches, for example, your waist size should be under 32 inches.

This also means that if you carry weight in your hips, there's nothing to worry about. It is crucial that no matter where you carry your weight, the need to be physically active and eat healthily is a matter of importance. Eating right and exercising leads to sustainable and healthy weight loss.

If you are worried about your weight or if you feel like you're obese, or you know you are obese and you want to do something about it, your first step is to speak to a doctor, dietician, or nurse so they can suggest more healthy eating habits, check your current state of health, and recommend the right physical activities to help you get started towards a journey of healthy weight and healthy body.

Chapter 3 - How Does Intermittent Fasting Work?

The primary thing you need to know about intermittent fasting is that it is not a diet. It is simply a method of regulating your eating times and your non-eating times. With intermittent fasting, you gain more benefits other than just losing weight. As discussed in earlier chapters, intermittent fasting brings you a host of health benefits including it being the easiest eating routine you can follow.

While plenty of us are worried if we would have enough willpower to get through 16 hours or even 12 hours of fasting, once you look at it as a lifestyle choice rather than a 'Diet I need to go through because I want to lose weight', you would have already prepared your mindset to stick with the fast because essentially, you are not depriving yourself at all. The only limit you set yourself is consuming food at a certain time not limiting yourself to calorie intake or certain food groups.

Intermittent fasting is effective when you do it the right way, following the rules as well as exercising to increase its benefits.

Of course, it is still advised that you opt for healthier meal choices, such as lean meats, proteins, and vegetables during your meal times, but again the beauty of this method is that the choice is entirely yours. When you feel like it, it's alright to indulge in your favorite foods every now and again. There's no restriction and complete freedom.

What you're most likely to struggle with, especially in the early stages, is the hunger that you feel when you skip a meal. Like everything else, this change is going to take some getting used to before your body will adapt, and in the beginning, it can feel difficult to get through your daily tasks as you normally would because you would be focused on that hungry feeling.

The urge to want to binge and give in to your cravings can also be high in the early stages, which is something a lot of beginners also struggle with. That inner monologue of *it's okay, I can indulge in a little extra because I skipped a meal today* can be the devil on your shoulder that's hard to ignore.

Intermittent Fasting Protocols

Intermittent fasting involves switching the feasting and fasting cycles and this usually involves short-term fasts. Plenty of people fast for short periods of time to control their calorie intake. Most importantly, intermittent fasting also helps regulate the hormones that are connected to weight control. We will look into the benefits of intermittent fasting in a different chapter, but for now, let us first look at the different methods of fasting and see which one works best for you.

There are three popular methods to intermittent fasting which gives you flexibility in planning your approach. Having options is a great thing because it helps you switch things up but also helps you stick to something just because it works for you. Think about how many times in your life when you found you were more inclined to stick to something because there were options presented to you? If one method was not working out quite like you hoped it would, you always had the choice of choosing another way which would suit you better. You were not giving up on your goal, you were simply utilizing the options that you had to find the best possible way to reach that goal.

The three methods in which you can approach the intermittent fasting method are divided into either days or weeks, length of time, and duration between each fast. No longer will you have to be confined to just one way of having to lose weight. And why should you be when there are several options right in front of you to help you achieve that very same goal?

The different methods of intermittent fasting will each come with their own pros and cons, and you may need to experiment with them to find which pattern of eating is going to work best for you and your body type. When you are fasting, you are either going to be eating very little, or eating nothing at all, that would depend on the type of method you are going to choose. Without further ado, let us get right into exploring the different methods of intermittent fasting that await you.

In a nutshell, these methods are:

1. The 16/8 Method: You skip the most important meal of the day and only consume food during the 8-hour feasting window which is from 12noon to 8 pm.
2. The Eat-Stop-Eat: Each week, you commit to doing one or two 24-hour fast. So you do not eat a meal from dinner time today till dinner time the next, for example.
3. The 5:2 Diet: You only commit to consuming 500-600 calories for at least two or three days of the week but you go back to regular eating periods the rest of the four days.
4. The Warrior Diet: Involves fasting for 20 hours and have a 4-hour eating period. People who follow this diet usually eat one huge meal a day.

The major rule here is that you do not compensate by consuming more calories during your fasting window. Now, let us look into more detail what each of the methods is about.

- **The 16/8 Method**

This method also goes by another name – the Leangains method. If you choose to go with this option, what is going to happen is that you will need to skip your breakfast each morning, thereby restricting your daily window eating opportunity periods to just 8 hours per day. For example, the timeframe at which you will be able to eat could be from 1 pm – 9 pm at night, and after 9 pm (your cut-off time), you will not be fueling your body with any more food for the next 16-hours.

16-hours is the recommendation for men to go by, and for women, it is 14-hours because men and women's bodies work differently. During your periods of fast, it is important that you do not consume any calories at all. If you feel that nagging feeling to have something, diet soda, sugar-free gum, black coffee, and calorie-free sweeteners are some options that you could consider. Alternatively, chew on a celery stick. It has zero calories!

The easiest way to get accustomed to this method is to simply have your fast at night because that is when you will be sleeping anyway and not likely to consume any calories during that time. Once you wake up in the morning, all you would have to do is wait six hours and you can start eating again.

This method is among the most flexible, which can easily be adapted to suit your lifestyle, but keeping it consistent is the key to seeing results. If it isn't kept consistent, you risk throwing your hormones completely off balance, which will make it much harder for you to stick to the program and see any visible results. It is also important to note that the times when you can eat does not mean that you can gorge on anything you want. What you eat is still going to matter if you want to lose weight on this program, and it is important to choose healthy and wholesome meals.

If you are exercising on the days that you are intermittent fasting, it is advisable to consume more carbs on that day so your body has more fuel to burn. Protein consumption should also be high daily, although this would vary depending on your age, gender, body fat, type of daily activities, and your personal goals.

The good: This is flexible enough to be adapted to suit your needs. You can still eat your favorite foods (in moderation) during your eating timeframes and not have to deprive yourself of the simple pleasures in life.

The not-so-good: The guidelines of what you can and cannot eat can be pretty specific, placing emphasis on only nutritious meals, especially if you are planning to work out on that day. Scheduling your meals around your workout days can be a challenge to stick to.

- **The 5:2 Method**

This one involves eating only 400-500 calories but only on two non-consecutive days per week. The other 5-days? You get to eat like you normally would (in moderation, of course). This method is easy enough to follow; all you have to do is technically eat very little on one day, and eat normally the next day. The average woman should ideally consumer about 2,000 to 2,500 calories per day respectively, but on this method, you're only going to be consuming a maximum of 500 calories on your intermittent fasting diet days.

The good: Meal replacement shakes can make this method easier to cope with on your low-calorie days, and they still have the essential nutrients that you need. Meal replacement shakes should not be used frequently, only during the initial stages when you're easing your body into the process.

The not-so-good: The temptation to binge-eat on your regular meal days is the danger that comes with this method. Tracking and planning your meals will help ensure that you don't fall into the trap of overeating, which will make your low-calorie days pointless if you gain the calories back during those 5-days of eating normally.

• The Eat-Stop-Eat Method

On this method, you are going to be fasting for 24-hours and only doing so either once or twice a week. This means that if your last meal of the day was dinner, you would not be eating anything throughout the entire next day until it is time for dinner again. No food can be consumed during this 24-hour window, although you can make use of the little loophole and treat yourself to some calorie-free beverages if you want (best not to, of course!).

Once the 24-hour window is up, you can go back to eating normally. This method helps to reduce the calories you are consuming overall, without leaving you feeling like you are limiting the food that you eat. Technically, you are not depriving yourself of the foods you still like, you're just limiting how often and when you consume them. Regular workouts are still going to be important to maintain weight loss and keep it off.

The good: If you have never done this before, 24-hours can seem like an awfully long time to go without food, but the good thing is that this plan is flexible. This is not an all-or-nothing method. If you're just starting this, try going for as long as you can without food while you let your body adjust to the new regime. A good tip will be to start this method on a day when you're swamped with work and unlikely to have time to be thinking about food.

The not-so-good: 24-hours of not eating could be too much for some people to handle. Some symptoms of food deprivation may occur, which include fatigue, headaches, anxiety, or just plain cranky, although it does get better over time as your body starts to get used to it. Self-control is the biggest challenge of this method.

The 20-Hour Fast (the Warrior Diet)

The Warrior Diet is a type of structured diet that involves a fasting period of 20 hours followed by a feasting period of 4 hours and the name is derived from nutritional habits of warriors who weren't in the habit of eating 3 or even 6 meals a day. Warriors from the Roman cultures to Spartan elite warriors lived on an average of one or two large meals, usually one in the evening and one in the morning.

This diet has been criticized as not being a true type of intermittent fasting. The reason for this is the time between both meals which is about a minimum of 8 to a maximum of 10 hours between feeding yourself during dinner and during breakfast. The time is not long enough to reap the benefits of tasting.

Apart from that, this type of fasting also allows small consumption of foods. You are able to eat mild servings of raw fruits and vegetables or even a few servings of protein. For those practicing this type of diet, they have foregone small meals and just have one huge warrior meal.

The good: This 20-hour fast enables you to reap the benefits of increased growth hormone. This type of fasting also results in fewer calories consumed, provided you stick to the 1 meal a day ratio. With this diet, you have one large meal and the make-up of the meal is not a huge concern. Dieters using this fast usually create 'junkier' foods for their one-big meal. For those with lack of time, having one meal a day makes like simpler.

The not-so-good: The drawback in the Warrior Diet exists in other fasts as well. This drawback is about the meal itself- having to get all your essential calories and nutrients into ONE meal. This means this one big meal is going to be a huge meal and this can often lead to discomfort. But you can always combat this by ensuring that you focus on wholesome foods from calories, veggies, and rice so you meet at least 2,000 calories. You can't get them from chicken wings and fries.

Which Method is right for me?

Ultimately, it would depend on you and what your body will be able to handle. No two people are built in exactly the same way, especially not men and women and the results are going to vary dramatically because of that. Some people might experience success with one method, while others might find what they're looking for in another.

The point of intermittent fasting is to reduce the *number* of calories that your body is consuming. The lower the intake, the better the weight loss, and provided that you don't compensate for this by eating too much during the days where you can eat, weight loss should happen.

Those who have tried this method have found the 16/8 intermittent fasting method one of the easiest out of all the options because you can do this while you're sleeping. because when Intermittent fasting leads to fat loss your body is in a state where it is fed, it is digesting and absorbing the food which is coming into the body.

Each fed state will last approximately three to five hours as your body works to digest and absorb all the food you have just eaten, and in this state, it is hard for your body to burn off the excess fat because your insulin levels will be high.

Once the fed state has come to pass, your body will then move into a post-absorptive state, which is when it is not working to process any food at all. This can last for up to 8 to 12 hours after the last meal that you had, and this is when you are going into the *fasted* state. Here, it becomes much easier for your body to then burn fat because your insulin levels are much lower, and your body can work to burn the fat that was previously inaccessible to it during its fed state.

Intermittent fasting is effective because without this method, very rarely do our bodies get the opportunity to enter the fasted state it needs to burn fat. Not only will this method help you achieve weight loss, but you have the option of doing it without changing much about what you eat, how often you exercise, or how much you eat (again, don't overdo it).

How can I decide which method works for me?

Here are a few things you can try to figure out which would suit you best:

- **Look at your eating patterns.** Which meal do you consume the most calories and which meals do you consume the least? Identifying this would help you eliminate one meal time and this would be ideal for the 16/8 method.

- **Look at your daily schedule.** Do you work out? What time do you work out? Which part of your day are you most active? While plenty of people skip breakfast with the 16/8 method, maybe you can't because you work out in the morning? Or you need the energy to commute to work, taking buses, trains, and trams. So maybe you can have your breakfast and lunch but skip dinner. Or what if you're not active at all? Then perhaps the 5:2 Method works since it can help you can reduce your calories.

- **Look at your weekly schedule.** Maybe the only time when you can actually go on a fast is on weekends? Because every other day is packed with exercise, meetings, commuting and going to and from one location to another and you just need the energy from food? Then only during the weekends can you take a break and give your mind, your soul as well as your body a break? You don't do work, you take time to relax, and you can go on a fast to give your digestive system a break.

- **Trying all of them.** You can switch up your feasting and fasting patterns to identify which works best. If you want to do this, you must give adequate time in between these methods. It is unhealthy to do a 16/8 fast one day and two days later do a 24-hour fast and then 4 days later switch to a 5:2 fast. You mess up your hormones as well as your mind. If you want to try each of these methods, commit to each for at least a month before moving on to the next method. This will give you a better gauge of what works for your daily schedule, your weekly schedule as well as your eating patterns.

Chapter 4- Intermittent Fasting, The Best Anti-Aging Agent

Who doesn't love anti-aging solutions? We all want to slow down the aging process and at the very heart of anti-aging research and development, plenty of high-profile celebrities, entrepreneurs, and just about anyone wanting to stay young use intermittent fasting to combat aging.

In this chapter, we will look into the mechanism that creates the benefits of anti-aging and longevity. This chapter could be more scientific than the other chapters but it will attempt to zero in on the crucial details in an easy-to-understand format. By the end of this chapter, you will have a deeper understanding of the amazing benefits of intermittent fasting and its connection towards anti-aging.

Fasting Diets: The Difference between Micro-Fast vs Multi-Day Fasting

Before we focus on the aspects of intermittent fasting and its relation to healthy aging, it is crucial to understand the difference between multi-day fasting as well as micro fasting.

These differences are important to recognize because they provide context.

Short-term fasting protocols, which are a form of intermittent fasting, are a period of time-restricted eating where no calories are consumed for at least 16 to 20 hours and they have amazing benefits. These micro-fasts also support better metabolic functions by improving our glycemic control and also lowering insulin levels. What's great about this is that it also helps our body control weight!

Short-term fasting for weight loss may be an extremely credible and sustainable lifestyle choice. According to some studies, the fat mass goes down during fasts whereas physical strength is unchanged. Apart from the above, the other benefits of micro-fasting are also related to cardiovascular support and an increased brain-derived neurotrophic factor (BDNF) which provides a signal to the brain.

Also, nightly fasting of 13 hours also has shown to lower the risks of cancer.
When it comes to prolonged-fast, this is usually over a period of 48 hours to trigger various physiological changes that connect to unique fasting benefits that relate to functional areas such as longevity, immune strength, and healthy aging.

A study done in 2014 in Cell magazine explains the difference between micro and prolonged fasting. This explanation says that the physiological changes resulting from prolonged-fasting are more pronounced than the ones as a result of micro-fasting or time-restricted fasting less than 24 hours because of the requirements to change from a fat and ketone bodies based catabolism after the glycogen reserves are reduced.

This study also found that when a person went through prolonged fasts, the body increases its white blood cells and it is also a useful adjunct therapy that is used alongside chemotherapy for killing cancer cells. A good rationale behind this study is that cancer cells grow and love glucose so by going through prolonged fasts, we starve these cancer cells and support the efforts of anti-cancer immunes.

How does Intermittent Fasting promote Anti-Aging?

The foundation of intermittent fasting is restricting everyday food intake to a six to eight-hour eating window and you fast for the rest of the time. The effects of fasting, apart from losing weight, are also to reduce the feeling of being hungry and to reduce the risk of chronic diseases from heart diseases and diabetes.

The body typically uses carbohydrates as fuel for a quick energy boost. But, when the body is starved of this resource and carbs are not available immediately, the body then looks for other types of energy sources such as fat. During the fasting window, the body transforms to a fat-burning state to ensure it gets its energy one way or another. When intermittent fasting is correctly done, it helps increase the body's energy levels and you also get better quality sleep.

A study conducted by Japanese and published in Scientific Reports has gone on to further investigate the effects of fasting on the human body by looking at individuals who have fasted for 58 hours. These individuals were analyzed for their whole plasma, blood as well as red blood cells. What did the study find? The study found that a long period of fast boosted the metabolic rate of these individuals, it generated antioxidants, and it also had anti-aging effects.

The research also identifies 44 metabolites, where 30 of them were unreported substances that increased significantly during fasting. Three metabolites which are leucine, ophthalmic as well as isoleucine increased during a fast and these metabolites were known to lessen aging effects.

These three metabolites are crucial in the maintenance of muscle as well as antioxidant activity. This research suggests that when we fast, it helps promote the production of these metabolites thus increasing the rejuvenating effect and longevity.

Also, compounds purine and pyrimidine which play a crucial role in protein synthesis and gene expression was also seen to be more evident. This enhanced metabolism not only boosts the body's antioxidant production but also promotes optimized cell functions. Increased antioxidant production also helps protect cells from free radicals during metabolism. When individual fasts for over 58-hours, these antioxidants increase significantly.

Fasting may boost production of age-related metabolites

Based on the research by these Japanese scientists, we now know that boosted production of age-related metabolites can be enhanced even in older individuals through fasting. This means fasting is not only focused on just losing weight, but it can also be effective against the signs of aging as well as from eliminating the threat of free radicals by increasing the antioxidant metabolites.

So, if weight loss is not your goal, you may want to try intermittent fasting anyway as a method to combat aging symptoms and also promote a lifespan that has fewer radicals. Maintaining a calorie balanced together with healthy weight and regulating insulin are all the amazing benefits of intermittent fasting. When you do this, you're not only hitting one goal, you are hitting plenty of various healthy goals along your path towards a sustainable and healthy weight loss.

Chapter 5- Intermittent Fasting - The Good & The Bad

Weight loss is almost everyone's primary goal, especially if you're a woman. That's the reason many ventures on a diet, isn't it? Because they want to lose weight, although there are some who are doing it for the other health benefits that go along with a diet. The beauty of intermittent fasting is it's one – and possibly – the easiest "diet" routine to follow because it isn't really a diet at all. Not in a conventional sense anyway.

Diets normally incur cutting out certain types of food or minimizing your calorie intake to a restrictive amount, which makes those types of diets difficult to stick to for the long-term because you're depriving your body that never is a pleasant feeling. Often it takes immense amounts of willpower, commitment, and dedication to stick to a diet for years, and many fall off the wagon along the way and go back to their old eating habits because deprivation only leads to cravings. If you've ever experienced that before, you'll know how hard it is to keep the cravings at bay, which is why most of the diets these days are ineffective.

And that's what makes intermittent fasting *so* effective because you're not depriving yourself at all. This method requires forgoing one meal a day, but it doesn't limit you to only consuming certain food groups when it does come time for you to eat. In fact, go ahead and eat what you normally would (but don't overdo it of course!), and combined with exercise, it will still be effective in helping you lose weight and belly fat because skipping one meal a day already equals fewer calories than what you would normally consume.

Of course, it is still advised that you opt for healthier meal choices, such as lean meats, proteins, and vegetables during your meal times, but again the beauty of this method is that the choice is entirely yours. When you feel like it, it's alright to indulge in your favorite foods every now and again. There's no restriction and complete freedom.

General Benefits of Intermittent Fasting

Do you want to know why intermittent fasting could be the ideal weight-loss method for you? Especially when you've got a busy and hectic schedule to contend with? It's because of the simplicity of this method, how it requires minimal effort on your part. Intermittent fasting is designed to fit into almost every lifestyle, even if you're always on the move. Here's why:

- **You Don't Spend Any Extra Time** – In fact, skipping one meal a day possibly even saves you time, because that 30 minutes to an hour which you spend on your meal could now be filled with other productive activities, which means you get more done during the day. You don't have to meal-prep as much when you're preparing one meal less, which also saves you time. Every little moment saved is a moment more that you could get more things done.

- **You're Able to Think Clearly** – Admit it, there have been several occasions where you've often felt sluggish at work, especially after a big meal. Not just at work, but at home too. That's because your body is busy digesting food, which causes you to feel more lethargic, making you feel less productive and like you could sleep for several hours. Which is why intermittent fasting is so great for mental clarity since when your body is not too preoccupied with digesting its meals, your mind is better able to focus on the task you have at hand. If you're currently trying the intermittent fasting and skipping lunch, you'll be able to see the difference for yourself, how there's no longer that sluggish, lazy feeling you get after eating. Instead, you feel focused, energized, and ready to power through to 5 pm.

- **It Saves You Money** – Eating one meal less means spending on one meal less, and that money can be redirected back into your savings account. You can even save money with groceries because the ingredients for your meals now last much longer when you're eating less than you normally would. When you look at how much you've been able to save at the end of the month just by cutting out one meal a day from your schedule, you'll be a lot more motivated to stick to this method even more than you already are.

- **It Helps You Lose Weight & Keep It Off** – Needless to say, this is probably one of the biggest physical benefits that most people would look forward to. It's not just about losing weight, equally important is keeping the weight off for good, which is why the intermittent fasting method is the only method that has proven to be able to do this. This goes back to the earlier point about not restricting yourself to only certain food groups and being able to eat regularly so you don't feel like you're depriving yourself in any way. The happier you feel about your diet and being able to eat the foods you like is the difference that makes intermittent fasting more effective than anything else out there.

- **You Become More Confident & Disciplined** – When you look good, you feel good, which is why people embark on a weight loss journey, isn't it? Because they want to look like the best version of themselves. Intermittent fasting can do that for you, and not only will you end up looking and feeling much healthier, when you see how good you look in the mirror your confidence level increases. Your confidence levels will also be aided by the fact that intermittent fasting has taught you to be a more disciplined individual, focused on a goal, and being able to accomplish a goal that you set out to do. You need some level of discipline to succeed even with intermittent fasting because you need to be able to say no in the face of delicious food when it's not your time to eat. Sticking to a regular eating regimen helps to build your discipline levels, and when you can do that, your confidence levels are one again elevated because you can look back and say yes, I did it!

- **It Reduces Your Risk of Developing Type 2 Diabetes** – Losing weight makes your body more insulin sensitive, which lowers your blood sugar levels. Eating makes our bodies release insulin into the bloodstream so that it can supply our cells with the energy we need. However, those who are already pre-diabetic will already be insulin-resistant, which means their blood sugar levels remain elevated, and that's why going on the intermittent fasting method could go a long way in helping this. Fasting means your body would need to produce insulin less often because you're not consuming any food, which could help to stabilize your insulin secretion.

- **It Reduces Your Risk of Cardiovascular Disease** — Fasting is not the same as starvation. You're not cutting yourself off from food completely, you're simply eating less. Minimizing your calories will help to minimize your risk of cardiovascular disease because by losing weight, you simultaneously reduce your blood pressure levels, lower your cholesterol and triacylglycerol levels, all of which help to keep heart disease at bay.

Health Benefits of Intermittent Fasting

- **Faster Metabolism**

We have touched this aspect earlier in the book. A healthy metabolism is very important for an active body. If your metabolism is working fine, it is much easier for you to lose weight and fight other health issues. You would feel more energetic and lively with the help of an active metabolism.

However, this can become a problem when you start reducing your calorie intake below a certain level.

Whenever you decide to lower your calorie intake for a prolonged period, your body ends up lowering the metabolic rate to avoid over expenditure energy. This would be a big hurdle not only in losing weight but also in leading a healthy life. While it is going to be important in helping preserve your life if there was a lack of food, it is going to stop you from losing weight.

There is no risk of slowing metabolism by following intermittent fasting. Your body never faces a shortage of calories within a day. It only stops receiving calories for a specific time interval and then gets the regular number of calories.

This temporary shortage and then restocking of calories never allow the metabolic rate to slow down. You will always feel the same amount of energy, vigor, and vitality while you follow intermittent fasting. Once your body gets adapted to ketosis and starts burning fat, you will feel more energetic as fat fuel is cleaner and long-lasting. There would be no sudden bursts of energy like you experience when you are taking a high carbohydrate diet.

Studies have shown that Short-term fasts followed in intermittent fasting can increase your metabolism by 14%. It will give a great boost to your weight loss efforts.

- **Better Cognitive Function**

Some people argue that fasting would affect their cognitive functioning. The brain needs a lot of glucose all the time to function. Yes, it is a fact that your brain needs a lot of energy all the time to function. It is the most energy-hungry organ in the body. However, following an intermittent fast has no adverse effect on the functioning of the brain.

The brain is undoubtedly the most pampered organ of the body. The whole body is actively trying to protect and nurture it. The primary fuel used by the brain is glucose, but it can also run from the energy provided by ketones. So, even if you are not eating anything for a few days, your brain would keep working smoothly.

Studies have proven that brain function can actually improve after a short interval of fasting. Studies have also shown that intermittent fasting can also help in reversing the progression of several neurodegenerative diseases like Alzheimer's and

Parkinson's disease. It increases neuroplasticity and helps in the regrowth of nerve cells.

It increases the production of a special stimulator known as Brain Derived Neurotropic Factor (BDNF) by 50-400%. This BDNF is the main stimulator that increases neuroplasticity, and the brain can actively reproduce the lost never cells that lead to problems.

- **Build Muscle Mass While You Lose Fat**

Building muscle is comparatively easy while you are following intermittent fasting. There is a strong reason that the bodybuilding community all around the globe is actively following intermittent fasting.

Intermittent fasting helps in bulking muscles while you cut down body fat. People have a misconception that when the body gets short of glucose energy, it starts burning muscle protein. The body does burn some protein, but that is only the unstructured protein present in your blood. It wouldn't start eating muscles in such a short span. It would get counterproductive.

When you start doing intermittent fasting, your body releases a lot of hormones that promote faster muscle growth and also cause fat loss. Several intermittent fasting protocols have great potential for bulking muscles and reducing the body fat ratio.

- **Normalize Your Blood Sugar Levels**

High blood sugar levels are a big cause of health disorders. They cause diabetes and also chronic inflammation and stress. If the blood sugar levels remain consistently high, then the body wouldn't be able to function smoothly — the risk of diseases like cardiovascular damage, high blood pressure, and stroke increases manifold.

Therefore, keeping high blood sugar levels under check is important. At present, more than 100 million people in the US are either facing diabetes or pre-diabetes which will, later on, turn into diabetes. Insulin resistance is at the back of the problem, and intermittent fasting is one of the best ways to improve insulin sensitivity for normalized blood sugar levels. At least for people suffering from Type II Diabetes, intermittent fasting is a great boon. It can help them in living a healthy life free from the dangers of diabetes.

- **Improve Insulin Sensitivity**

Intermittent fasting helps your body in reversing insulin resistance. We have already discussed that insulin resistance is the primary cause of most health issues and also a reason for uncontrolled weight gain. By following intermittent fasting, you can eliminate the main reason for developing insulin resistance.

The greater the amount of time your body remains without the release of further insulin, the better will be the insulin sensitivity. This is one thing that gets possible only when you are in a fasted state bringing insulin sensitivity while frequent eating isn't practically possible. However, if you put even a little bit of control over your eating habits and shorten your eating windows, you can develop insulin sensitivity.

It means you can reverse insulin resistance and bring insulin sensitivity without doing anything else at all. No medication, no exercise, or any other measure will be required. This can be among the biggest health gains you could have. Improved insulin sensitivity will help you in losing weight and also in improving the overall health biomarkers. The chronic inflammation and stress in your body would also go down as insulin resistance is primarily behind these problems.

- **Improve Stress Response**

Chronic stress is a big problem for all of us. The modern life is so hectic that we always remain under stress. There is so much competition, and aspirations are so high that they also keep us in stress. However, like with mental stress, there is also physiological stress that your body experiences all the time due to internal issues.

For instance, insulin resistance can cause adrenal stress in your body. When the insulin levels in the blood remain high, the adrenal gland in your body starts releasing the stress hormone called 'Cortisol.' The function of this hormone is to ease the body functions. However, if the levels of the stress hormone are high and they remain consistent, then it can also push your body towards weight gain.

The presence of cortisol in the blood is a sign that the body is under stress, and hence, it gets defensive. It stops all the new regeneration work and chronic inflammation starts taking over. High blood pressure and liver issues are also very common due to high physiological stress. This can push your body very hard. The chronic stress is behind most cardiovascular injuries and strokes.

Your body is not used to the stress, and whenever there is a surge, it causes severe problems. Intermittent fasting can help you in addressing this problem to a great extent. It has a two-way approach to stress. First, intermittent fasting helps in resolving the issues that lead to chronic stress. It promotes insulin sensitivity, decreases chronic inflammation, and helps in normalizing the blood pressure and sugar levels besides helping in other problems.

Second, intermittent fasting in itself puts your body through mild stress. This helps your body in getting used to this stress. So, in case of an eventuality where the body goes through acute stress, the reaction wouldn't be knee-jerk. Even most of the ischemic heart injuries have sudden stress at their back. Improving stress response by putting the body under some mild-positive stress is a great help that you can get from intermittent fasting.

- **Boost HGH Levels**

Human Growth Hormone (HGH) is a very powerful hormone produced by your body. As the name suggests, the main function of this hormone is to promote growth. It is the primary hormone responsible for the building of muscles, tissues, bones, and overall growth. Our body produces this hormone in high quantities during childhood as the growth demands are high.

The production reaches its peak while we reach puberty. However, once you cross the teenage, the production of this hormone starts slowing down. You stop growing and hence the body doesn't feel the need to produce this hormone.

However, this is the time when you start experiencing the downward spiral of aging. HGH is a hormone that rapidly helps in regeneration of cells and tissues. It keeps your skin tight and makes healing faster. It is truly a wonder hormone. Somehow, if the natural production of HGH remains very high, a person may not experience aging as we do. It also keeps your immune system very high. It is also the main fat-burning hormone.

Our body doesn't even stop producing HGH, but the production remains limited. HGH is released in short bursts and that too under special conditions.

Under normal circumstances, the HGH production is the highest when:

1. Your stomach is empty.
2. The insulin levels in the blood are very low.

3. You are sleeping.

The best way to take maximum advantage of HGH is to do high-intensity interval training before ending your fast as the HGH levels will be the highest at that time. The HGH will help your body in burning fat and building muscle as these are the two main functions of this hormone. Our body also releases HGH in high quantities when you experience any major injury or trauma. This happens as your body's need for reconstruction is high, and it also needs protection.
Normally, the three conditions mentioned above are the best for increasing HGH. Intermittent fasting helps in the creation of all these conditions and boosts the production of HGH in the body.

While you are practicing intermittent fasting, your stomach becomes empty after a short period as the food gets digested and the new intake of food isn't initiated. You remain in the fasted state for much longer for instance 16 hours. It gives a lot of time to your body to produce HGH.

The intermittent fasting also helps in lowering the insulin levels in your blood. It promotes insulin sensitivity, and hence your insulin levels start remaining under control. Even if you still have insulin resistance, the levels would anyhow go down after

8-12 hours of your last meal. This means your body will still get at least 4-8 hours for producing HGH in ideal condition.

It is always the best to remain in the fasted state at night as time passes faster in sleep and you feel less inclined to eat. This also fulfills the remaining condition facilitating the production of HGH. Studies have proven that intermittent fasting can increase the production of HGH in women by 1,400%. This percentage can go as high as 2000% in men. If you are doing high-intensity exercise in the fasted state, then these levels of HGH can go even higher.

The whole world, especially the people involved in bodybuilding and performance sports are crazy behind this hormone. The demand is so high for the hormone that people are ready to pay exorbitant prices for the synthetically produced HGH illegally. Using a synthetic version is wrong as it has more side effects than advantages.

You can boost the production of HGH in your body through intermittent fasting.

- **Lower Chronic Inflammation**

Inflammation is our body's natural reaction to any damage. It is a protective system that directs the body's protective mechanism to the affected area. However, if inflammation in any particular area, organ, or system persists for very long, it can start acting against the body itself. Such inflammation is called chronic inflammation, and it is a silent danger.

Chronic inflammation in any area of the body can aggravate the problem. It will keep nullifying the body's attempt to treat the problem. It will weaken the immune system and also hamper the functioning of that particular organ or system. Chronic inflammation can take place in any area and cause great havoc. For instance, if chronic inflammation takes place in the fat cells, the victim's body would never be able to have any control over the amount of food he/she eats. It is a common problem in people suffering from obesity. The fat cells in their body should send a signal to the brain that the fat stores are ample and there is no need to consume more food.

However, inflammation in the fat cells causes the hormones from the fat cells to break loose, and this creates resistance in the brain towards the signals. Their body keeps sending the signal that eating must be stopped, but they can't resist food. It isn't their love for food but a miscommunication of the hormonal system and the brain caused by inflammation.

Chronic inflammation degrades your body's inflammatory response. It leads to damage to healthy cells, tissues, and organs. If untreated, this can even lead to DNA damage, tissue death, and internal scarring. Several diseases like cancer, heart problems, rheumatoid arthritis, type 2 diabetes, obesity, Alzheimer's, and asthma also spread fast if one had chronic inflammation. Intermittent fasting helps your body in fighting chronic inflammation. The positive processes initiated by intermittent fasting reduce the production of free fatty acids and the resultant oxidative stress. These are the main reasons for chronic inflammation. Healthy eating and better food choices can further help in the production of antioxidants that will help in fighting chronic inflammations. Therefore, it is a very reliable way of fighting chronic inflammation.

What Side-Effects (Cons) Can You Expect Should You Choose to Try This Diet?

If you're a woman, what you can expect is a possible hormonal imbalance, along with possibly disrupting your menstrual cycle because your body isn't consistently receiving the food that it has come to expect regularly. Hormonal imbalances triggered by intermittent – if you don't slowly ease into it, that is – could potentially cause difficulty sleeping, anxiety, and even depression, along with fertility issues if your menstrual cycle is affected because of the diet.

Which is why it is important for women to follow the recommendations of this fasting method and not try to do too much too soon.

Other possible side effects which you might experience, especially if this is your first time and you're not used to the fasting of any sort, include:

- Dizziness
- Fatigue
- Poor cognitive function, which is a common occurrence in the early stages
- Headaches
- An increase in cravings and the urge to binge (temptation can be strong, especially when you're just starting out)
- It could affect your regular exercise regime as you may not have the energy to push through your workouts, especially the high-intensity ones when you don't have as much energy to exert

What you're most likely to struggle with, especially in the early stages, is the hunger that you feel when you skip a meal. This is perfectly normal, because your body has already come to expect food, and a change in that schedule is bound to affect you. Like everything else, this change is going to take some getting used to before your body will adapt, and in the beginning, it can feel difficult to get through your daily tasks as you normally would because you would be focused on that hungry feeling.

The urge to want to binge and give in to your cravings can also be high in the early stages, which is something a lot of beginners also struggle with. That inner monologue of *it's okay, I can indulge in little extra because I skipped a meal today* can be the devil on your shoulder that's hard to ignore. But ignore it you must, because if you give in to your cravings, it defeats the whole purpose of intermittent fasting in the first place, since binge eating will probably end up with you consuming more calories than you normally would have.

Chapter 6 - The Women's Guide to Intermittent Fasting

No doubt you would be eager to get started on your intermittent fasting journey, especially after reading or hearing about the benefits that you stand to gain from it, weight loss especially. However, before you begin, there is one very important thing that needs to be highlighted – intermittent fasting works different for both men and women, and depending on your body type, it may not be for everyone.

Intermittent fasting for women can bring about the following benefits, which include:

1. Increasing your lean muscle mass
2. Long-term and sustainable weight loss
3. Improved energy levels
4. An increase in the production of the neurotrophic growth factor, which could help to provide relief for depression and even boost your cognitive function
5. Reduced levels of oxidative stress

Women also burn and store fat different from men. Women also lose weight differently from men. Therefore, intermittent fasting should also be done different because our bodies are so very different. Even amongst women, no two women are going to have the exact same bodies or bodily functions.

What makes the biggest difference is the hormones, specifically the human growth hormone (HGH), which is what helps women shed their excess body fat. Men naturally have higher levels of HGH than women do, which explains why they lose weight faster in general. If intermittent fasting is not done correctly for women, it could cause hormonal imbalance.

Despite the benefits that women stand to gain from intermittent fasting, women's bodies work on a whole different level compared to their male counterparts. When a woman's body senses that it is heading towards a state of famine, it will work to increase the production of the hormone responsible for hunger – known as leptin and ghrelin – which will signal to your brain that you're hungry and you need to eat. This is because women's bodies – thanks to the reproductive abilities – are more sensitive towards states of starvation and it immediately tries to protect itself from it.

This heightened level of sensitivity and the range of hormones in a woman's body is why intermittent fasting may not work as well for women if not done correctly. Hormone imbalance has a bigger implication on women than it does on men because of the way the female body is designed to create and carry life.

Additionally, because of the different hormones that women produce in their bodies, intermittent fasting could also potentially cause irregular periods, fertility issues, difficulty sleeping, anxiety, depression, and it could even cause your ovaries to shrink. Again, this is not necessarily true for everyone, but it could be the case for some.

Should Women Still Consider Intermittent Fasting Then?

The answer is yes. Like everything else, intermittent fasting is about finding the balance that works for you. Everything has got its pros and cons if you think about it, but if you can find that balance, the good will still outweigh the bad in the long run.

What women could do in this case is consider doing intermittent fasting at smaller timed intervals compared to men. Shorter faster periods could still prove to be beneficial if your goal is to lose weight and belly fat, without disrupting your hormones too much so the fasting method is still beneficial.

Again, the key to remember in this diet is about not going extreme right out of the gate. Yes, you're eager to lose weight and to start experiencing all the health benefits intermittent fasting promises, but you need to listen to your body at the same time.

Taking it one step at a time, slow, and steady is how you win the eventual race.

Here's a list of suggestions about how to make intermittent fasting work best for you as a woman:

- Drink plenty of fluids during your fast (water is the best)
- Fasting for 12-hours would be the right balance
- Never fast for longer than 24-hours at a time
- Do not fast on consecutive days, keep it at two to three days a week, especially in the beginning
- Lightweight exercises such as walking, stretching, and yoga would be a great add-on to your intermittent fasting days if you still want to get some exercise in there.
- Avoid intermittent fasting during pregnancy and if you're nursing.
- Avoid intermittent fasting if you're experiencing or undergoing chronic stress

- If you struggle with sleep disorders, avoid this fasting method for now

Why Intermittent Fasting for Women needs to be Different than Men?

Men and women are different. There are subtle differences that are not only physical but emotional and mental between the two genders. Therefore, measuring them both with the same yardstick can become problematic.

The biggest thing that makes treatment of women differently than men imperative is their ability to have children. This requires a special body and hormonal structuring and makes all the difference. Therefore, you can talk about all the equality, feminism, and all those things, but nothing should undermine the fact that women have a different physical and hormonal structure that needs special attention.

Women have been entrusted with the responsibility to bear kids. The whole process of bearing kids, making it, and providing the required nutrition is heavily dependent. A woman's body gets prepared to bear a child as soon as it hits puberty.

The body doesn't understand the legal restraints, and it always tries to remain in a state of readiness to bear kids. Until you hit menopause, either you want to have kids or not, your body would always try to attract fat so that whenever conception takes place, it can bear a healthy child. This need for readiness makes a substantial difference in the feeding needs of men and women.

Physiologically speaking, a woman's body has a higher body fat percentage than men. While a man may have an ideal essential body fat ratio of 3-5%, the women may have it anywhere between 10-13%. Even in athletes, male body fat ratio lies between 6-13% whereas female body fat ratio can be as high as 14-20%. In average body type men, the body fat ratio should fall between 18-24%.

This ratio in women is between 25-31%. The reason for showing these stats is simple. It is important for women to understand that having a little higher body fat ratio is not only normal but natural. This is how their bodies have been designed. All those women, who are obsessed with zero figures or other such dimensions, may put their natural body cycle at risk. Therefore, whenever a woman thinks of losing weight, this fact should be kept in mind.

Another thing that mandates that women have a different fasting schedule than men is their hormonal system. The hormonal cycle of women is highly sensitive to hunger signals. They are more sensitive to starvation, and their bodies are designed to bear kids, and that cannot be possible when there is a shortage of food. Therefore, longer and difficult fasts would hurt your fertility and childbearing abilities.

- This makes it necessary that women always move ahead with fasting schedules very slowly.
- They should never start with longer food gaps without practice.
- They must always increase their fasting period in small progression.
- They should not be adamant about continuing fasting for the complete duration. If there is a strong craving, they should end their fast that day and begin fresh the next day again.
- Women shouldn't keep fasts longer than 24 hours as that can seriously mess up their hormonal cycle.

If these things are followed, even women can follow intermittent fasting easily.

Effect of Fasting on the Hormonal System of Women

Fasting tells the body it isn't a good time for fertility. When you fast for long and your body starts having an energy deficit on a consistent level, it starts conserving energy for necessary functions and fertility is not one among them. This has been proven through several studies that prolonged fasting can lead to shrinking of ovaries. Besides, the same impact has been visible even in male subjects. However, it is important to clarify here that these experiments have only been conducted on mice. The induced fasting time was only of a few days, but on the life scale of mice, it could have meant fasting for much longer.

However, besides everything else, it is an undisputed fact that fasting for long is a problem for women. Several hormones get affected. The estrogen levels get messed up if the fasting is not done carefully or calorie restriction is carried out.

Here, it is again important to clarify that this imbalance can happen with any calorie restriction followed by women. It means regardless of the method followed like diet, calorie restriction, or intermittent fasting, such problems can arise if due attention is not paid to the process.

Imbalance in the hormonal levels can have a wide impact. The practitioners may face metabolic disorders, weight loss ability, mood, bone density, energy, cognitive function, anxiety, and stress levels all may get affected. Impact of starvation on various hormonal balances would be:

Impact of Estrogen Imbalance

- Low energy
- Poor heart health
- Infertility
- Poor glucose regulation
- Weight gain
- Reduced skin and hair health
- Poor cognitive function.'
- Decreased bone density
- Poor muscle tone

Imbalance can also trip the Cortisol levels in your body. It is the stress hormone. The impact would be:

- Sugar cravings
- Low energy
- Anxiety
- Fatigue

- Insomnia

Thyroid imbalance can also take place. It may lead to:

- Weight gain
- Brain fog
- Depression
- Anxiety
- Dry hair dry skin
- Irregular periods
- The feeling of cold or hot flashes

Fasting is a very healthy practice. Intermittent fasting is an even improvised version of fasting to eliminate the harmful things so that only beneficial things can be retained. However, incorrect observation of any procedure will lead to negative fallouts. Therefore, it is important that women should follow intermittent fasting in the right way and very carefully. They need to be more observant about the changes and never become lax in their approach.

Chapter 7 - Important Things for Women to Keep in Mind While Practicing Intermittent Fasting

The most important thing for women to do to become successful in their intermittent fasting pursuit is to avoid giving 'starvation signals.' It sends the body into panic mode all of a sudden. The production of hunger hormones shoots up, and the body fiercely starts protecting the fat. In such cases, losing fat would become very challenging.

You can avoid all this very easily by following the things given below:

Don't Test the Limits

You must never try to stretch the fasting too far. You have to fast and then give your body the time to recover. If you are beginning fasting, never fast on consecutive days. Always allow your body the time to recover.

Don't Fast Too Long

Initially, you should begin by creating safe gaps between your meals. Eliminate snacks. Then try to stretch the gap between the meals a bit. Always ensure that the highest amount of time spent without food is at the beginning of the fast. It means it is always better to begin fasts early in the evening as you will not feel hungry. Stretching your fast for too long in the morning wouldn't be a very bright idea. In any case, the fasting duration should be anywhere between 12-14 hours only. Several studies have shown that women get much better results with comparatively shorter fasts than men.

No HIIT on Fasting Days

High-intensity interval training is an energy-demanding activity. It should be avoided at all costs on the fasting days, especially if you are beginning your intermittent fasting. It can drain you and create strong energy demands.

No Fasting During the Menstrual Cycle

There is significant blood loss during the periods, and your body needs a lot of rest. Your hormones are also going crazy during this time. Therefore, you must not practice intermittent fasting at this time.

Have a Healthy Diet

Food choices are very important in the case of women as their nutritional requirements are high. You must choose a very healthy diet full of all the nutrients so that your hormones remain in check.

When To Stop

You should stop fasting if you notice the following things:

- Irregular periods or complete absence of periods
- Sudden resurfacing of sleep disorders without any apparent reason
- On facing sudden and drastic metabolic and digestive issues
- On experiencing sudden mood swings and brain fog
- On having sudden changes in the color of the skin or hair texture

Intermittent Fasting is NOT for You If:

- You have eating disorders
- Have got pregnant or trying to conceive
- Have sleep disorders
- Have adrenal fatigue
- You are suffering from PMS, PCOS, PCOD, Fibroids, Endometriosis, or other hormonal issues

Intermittent Fasting Lifestyle - The Things That Make It Different

Intermittent Fasting Isn't A Diet. It is a Routine.

Diets are restrictive; routines are liberating as they flow with life. You always find time to do things while following a routine as they are just a part of life. I don't believe people on diets would be able to say the same. So, it is very important that you make it clear in your mind that intermittent fasting isn't a diet. The biggest reason for diets to fail is that they put so many restrictions that people may or may not lose their weight, but they lose their peace of mind.

Imagine yourself at a party with people eating and merrymaking. Then imagine yourself standing in one corner sulking as you can't eat anything. Most of the food items that you like are there, but you can't have them. The steel-clad resolve of sticking to the diet flies out of the window that very moment. The people who can keep the resolve start developing a feeling of resentment.

Food is a very important requirement in life. It is needed for satisfying physical, mental, and emotional needs. Anything that is so restrictive cannot be adopted as a lifestyle.

Intermittent fasting, on the other hand, is very simple. You only need to remain in the fasted state for a set number of hours in a day or a week. The kind of diet you want to have, the amount of food you want to eat and the number of hours you want to spend doing an exercise can be up to your own choice. These will all help you in losing weight and staying healthier; however; you would still lose weight even if you don't eat the prescribed food items or don't sweat in the gym for long.

The biggest advantage of intermittent fasting is that it can be easily adopted as a lifestyle. You don't need to do anything out of the ordinary to follow intermittent fasting. You don't need to prepare elaborate meals. You don't need to be choosy every time you have to decide to eat something. Healthy eating is always advisable, but that doesn't mean you have to get extra picky.

Intermittent fasting is a very simple routine where you will have a certain number of hours in a day to eat. The remaining hours will be the fasting hours, and in them, you can't have anything besides the exempted items listed on the meal plan. The best thing is that after some time of practicing intermittent fasting, staying hungry for extra long wouldn't remain a problem at all.

It is more about when to eat and less about what or how much to eat

Intermittent fasting lays great emphasis on when to eat. The simple reasons for that are:

- Frequent meals cause great damage to our system as they keep our gut under constant pressure.
- The blood sugar levels remain consistently high as you keep eating food at short intervals.
- The insulin spike is also there, and hence, you remain prone to insulin sensitivity.
- It also increases cholesterol levels.
- Chronic inflammation also rises.
- Your body is not able to achieve satiety.
- Organs need to work extra hard to adjust the extra energy.

All this can be avoided by simply reducing the number of meals in a day. You don't need to reduce the number of calories you have in a day. You can still have your 2000 calories if you like. You can have even more if you want. You can also eat the pancakes once in a while and still lose weight because your body now has the time to focus on other things besides just digesting food.

The human body has passed through a long evolutionary process, and hence, it knows the processes that can help it run smoothly. The recent overexposure to food has complicated things a bit as the body not only gets busy in dealing with the extra energy, but it also has to deal with food items that are not very healthy. Once you start giving it the time to digest the food and begin the helpful processes, it can easily deal with the kind of food you eat.

Therefore, the real emphasis in intermittent fasting would always remain on maintaining the fasting state for a definite period in a day.

We can divide the day into two segments:

1. The Fasting Window: This is the time of the day during which you can't eat anything at all. There are some exceptions like unsweetened black tea or coffee, unsweetened fresh lime water or green tea that you can still have in this period as these don't add any calories or don't initiate your digestive process. Besides these items in limited quantity, you need to remain in a completely fasted state during this period. The fasting window is comparatively longer than the eating window. However, you can set the duration of the fasting window as per your convenience and tolerance.

2. The Eating Window: This is the time of the day during which you can eat. It is always advisable to have a smaller number of meals in a day. You must try to eliminate snacks and unnecessary munching as it leads to cravings and also causes insulin resistance, however, you can eat your fill in your eating windows. There are no calorie caps in intermittent fasting protocols. You need to make your meals as fulfilling as possible so that you don't feel the need to have snacks in between your meals. Healthy food items in the meals are always very good. They would help you in fighting obesity and chronic inflammation.

However, you can bring these changes one at a time, and there will not be a need to rush the process. The most important part of this to remember will always be to maintain fasting and eating windows.

Chapter 8 - What Works and What Doesn't in Intermittent Fasting

Intermittent fasting is a great way to stay healthy and burn fat. However, it is a process that needs to be carried out by you. Without your effort, even intermittent fasting cannot work. Certain things would increase the benefits of intermittent fasting and then there are others that would make your gains slowly. Therefore, you must know both types of things so that you can make an informed choice over things.

The Things That Work in Favor

Exercise

Exercise and especially, high-intensity interval training, works wonders if you are following intermittent fasting. The reason is simple; intermittent fasting boosts the production of hormones that can increase fat burn. High-intensity interval training creates the right environment at the right time. You may be engaging in high-intensity physical activity later in the day too. But, the effects wouldn't be the same as at that time, you would be in a fed state. In that case, there will be no presence of HGH in your bloodstream.

This is a hormone which can only be present when you are on an empty stomach after a long fasting interval. It acts as a very powerful steroid which is so potent that sports organizations have banned its use as it improves the performance of the athletes.

Therefore, exercise works in intermittent fasting. Not only high-intensity interval training but light cardio exercises, yoga, and aerobics also have their definitive health benefits. If you want to reap the full benefits of intermittent fasting, you must include exercise in your schedule.

Healthy Food

In this whole book, we have stressed the least on food. It has been intentional so that you can focus completely on the process and its advantages. However, this doesn't mean that food doesn't play an important role in fulfilling your objectives, or it isn't important.

First, healthy food is very important. You must try to consume as much fresh and unprocessed food as possible. Staying away from syrups, juices, jam, and jellies is always advisable as these things increase the number of calories consumed but don't give anything to your body. You must always avoid such things. Always eat fruits with their pulp. Throwing away the pulp and drinking only the juice is the biggest loss you will face ever.

Maintaining a balance among the macronutrients is also very important as reducing the number of meals consumed in a day also affects your calorie intake. If you do not have a balanced diet, you can get nutrient deficient.

Therefore, having a healthy diet helps in burning body fat and reducing weight.
If your goal specifically is fat burning, then you should take a keto diet along with intermittent fasting. Keto diet is a high-fat low-carb diet that helps your body in switching to burning fat fuel in place of glucose fuel. Once that process begins, fat burning becomes very fast and effective.

A Positive Attitude

Your attitude plays a very important role whenever bringing any change is considered. With a pessimistic attitude, a person may even lose hope of success or survival on falling even in a small pool. It is not the swimming skills that keep a person afloat but the will and confidence to survive. Recently, a Mexican survived in the Pacific Ocean for 438 days. No amount of swimming skills could have saved a person for that long in the Pacific. However, it was the optimism and will to survive that kept him alive.

Weight loss can get disappointing and disheartening at times. The reaction of people and over conscious attitude at times makes people look for faster results, and they don't follow procedure and then fail. Such things should never be taken to heart. You must always have confidence and the will to succeed. It is important that you keep making adjustments to get the desired results but looking for shortcuts can lead to failures. Health should always be a long-term goal as this is the only thing that matters in the end.

The Things That Work Against

Indiscipline

Indiscipline never works when it comes to any health goal. You can have some cheat days once in a while when you follow intermittent fasting and still expect results. However, you can't expect results by having some days of intermittent fasting once in a while when you treat all the days as cheat days. Intermittent fasting is a very relaxing process, and it doesn't impose severe restrictions on practitioners. However, the numbers of rules that are there have to be followed to get results.

Lack of Focus

It is important that you always remain focused on your goal. People keep losing focus while they follow any such things and then they complain that they aren't getting results. You will have to follow the eating and fasting windows, you will have to improve your eating habits, there should be a positive change in your food choices, and you must have a healthy exercise routine if you want to see quick results. You can't get results without focusing on the goal or putting efforts. Always remember 'There is No Free Lunch.'

Unhealthy Food

Intermittent fasting doesn't impose any strict dietary guideline for general practitioners. However, it may not tell things that you need to eat; there are certain things that you must not eat. If you are trying to lose weight, specifically eating the things that lead to weight gain are not going to help the cause. Therefore, it is important that you eliminate certain foods from your eating list.

Those food items are:

Refined Sugar: There is nothing else that would cause more obesity than refined sugar. It adds empty calories and causes inflammation in the liver cells. If your sugar consumption is high, avoiding food cravings would remain impossible for you. It is the first thing on the list that you need to eliminate. If you can't eliminate sugar, then you should make efforts to minimize its use.

Monosodium glutamate (MSG): It is a chemical that is used to add taste to food. It can cause chronic inflammation very fast. Soda, alcohol, and other sweetened beverages: all these things are high in sugar, and they add nothing to your digestive system. They raise your blood sugar levels, and hence, they must be avoided at all costs.

Fast Food and Processed Food: Fried and carb-rich food is a cause of most of the problems and obesity is at the top of them. You should sincerely try to avoid such foods. Even buying prepared salads from the stores is not a healthy option as they add salt, sugar, and preservatives for increasing sales. These things even make the salad unhealthy. The way to good health comes from healthy eating. You must keep it in mind while you follow intermittent fasting.

Chapter 9 - Transitioning to an Intermittent Fasting Routine

The right preparation is crucial for the success of any project, and your health cannot be any different. If any person embarks on the intermittent fasting journey and then leaves it feeling dejected, then there can be only one explanation, and that is starting without preparation.

Intermittent fasting would require fasting for unusually longer. Staying on the path may get difficult if you don't condition yourself properly. Our food habits are such that we consume a lot of sugar-rich foods. These food items lead to excessive cravings. If you are not preparing well, you will find it very difficult to remain in the fasted state.

Hunger pangs are another problem. Your hunger pangs are not an indication that your stomach is empty. Hunger pangs arise due to the release of a hormone called ghrelin. Your gut releases this hormone with clockwork precision. It means that if you are habitual of having snacks at 6 in the evening, then you would automatically start feeling hungry around six even if you had something an hour ago. You will need to learn to manage these hunger pangs too. Therefore proper preparation is very important.

Preparing Yourself for Intermittent Fasting

- **Eliminating Snacking Habits**

The current lifestyle has spoiled us all. We eat, as animals graze. It means there is no system of eating. There is no discipline or schedule. We can eat things simply because they are in front of us or someone else is eating them. There isn't any real correlation between eating and hunger anymore. This is a thing that's causing the problem. The greater the number of meals we have in a day, the faster we spin the wheel of insulin resistance and chronic inflammation. The higher the meal frequency we have, the more difficult it will be for us to bear hunger. The hunger pangs would be quicker.

The first thing you need to do is manage the number of meals you have in a day. If you look closely, almost 5-6 times in a day, we eat without any real purpose, and for 3-4 times, we eat for real reasons. This makes 10-11 meals a day. When you are feeling surprised that you've never had 10-11 meals in a day, hold your horses. Physiologically, any incident that spikes your blood sugar levels is a meal. It means if you had three soda cans in a day at three instances, then those are three meals. Even having a sweet, creamy coffee is also a meal for your body as the blood sugar levels increased nonetheless.

The normal day in the life of a person is:

1. Day starts with a Tea or Coffee   : 6-8 am
2. Breakfast   : 8-10 am
3. Morning Snacks   : 10-11 am
4. Lunch   : 1-3 pm
5. Evening Snacks   : 3-4 pm
6. Late Evening Snacks of Refreshments   : 5-7 pm
7. Dinner   : 8-10 pm
8. Post Dinner Snacks/ Sweets/ Coffee   : 10-11 pm

These are straight meals and snacks. I have discounted the number of times people munch sweet chewing gum, soda, tea, coffee, beer, and other things that increase your blood sugar levels. If this is a schedule with which you can relate to, then you will need to do a lot of restructuring and preparation is important for you.

Even before starting or planning to fast, you will need to reduce the number of meals you have in a day. Your first step should be to eliminate all kinds of snacks from your life. This wouldn't happen with some magic trick, will power, or determination. These things don't work in the long run. Everyone has weak moments. You can only do something reasonable when you cut the need for food.

You can only eliminate the need for snacks by having heavy fulfilling meals that help you in going from one meal to another without creating a gap for craving.
If you are not eating a healthy meal full of the right mix of macronutrients, it is very unlikely that you wouldn't feel hungry. Fat and protein are the things that keep you feeling full. If you had a high-fat breakfast, it is unlikely that you would need snacks around 10-11 am. However, if you simply had corn flakes or cereals for breakfast, snacks would become a necessity.

The reason is very simple, such breakfast is high in carbs, and hence, it burns fast and leads to hunger pangs. Therefore, correcting your meal and bringing a balance is crucial for making it through the day without facing hunger pangs and cravings.

- **Managing With Fewer Meals**

Once you have eliminated the snacks from your meals, it would be easier for you to begin any fast. The mantra would always be a healthy diet full of all the macronutrients. The next piece of the puzzle is to remain hungry for prolonged periods. This is a thing that comes out of practice.

It has been already discussed that hunger pangs are necessarily not a result of your body's need for food. There is a mechanism in your body that keeps reminding you to refill your body after a set interval of time. This process was very useful in the past when we had no way to know about time or had to make elaborate preparations to bring food to the table. However, things are very different these days. You can get food simply by calling the food providers. You can go out and eat. You can easily cook. But, the body has learned some things over millions of years of the evolutionary process, and it can't unlearn those things swiftly, and hence, you will have hunger pangs.

But, like a pet, you can control your hunger pangs. It is very easy and effective. You would need first to create gaps between your meals. Eliminate all the snacks from your routine. This will train your gut not to demand food between meals. Once you have achieved that, you should start creating an equal gap between your meals. It means if you are having three meals in a day, you should have them at almost equal intervals and at fixed times.

Within a few days, you will find that you have stopped experiencing hunger at other times. In the beginning, when you experience hunger other than the meal timings, you will have to bear those hunger pangs for a bit, and the hunger would subside. The ghrelin release is always very short, and it is easy to suppress.

The crucial part of the preparation involves limiting your meals to three or less. Then you should try to finish all these meals within a gap of 12 hours and have nothing for the remaining 12 hours. It isn't difficult at all as for the rest of the 12 hours, you will be full and sleeping for most of the time. There will be no problem in carrying out this part.

Once you have achieved this objective, you will be ready to begin intermittent fasting.
The following chapters will explain the various intermittent fasting protocols that you can follow. You can pick the fasting protocols as per your tolerance and health goals. When you prepare well and more in a focused way, you will get success very fast.

Things to Expect on Your Intermittent Fasting Journey

Intermittent fasting is a lifestyle change, and hence, you must expect some changes in the way you are leading your life. It is always wise to expect that you will have to make some minor corrections in your day to day activities.

When we talk of lifestyle change, it is important that you consider all the aspects of life, eating is just one of them. You will have to change your eating habits. Of late, it has become as if we are living to eat and not eat to live. Food is a primary necessity of life, but it is not the end goal. Living a healthy life that helps you in achieving meaningful goals should be your aim.

- **Eating Habits**

Eating habits, in general, have changed drastically in the past. The food-producing industry has contributed a lot to it. There have been aggressive marketing campaigns about eating smaller but frequent meals. Even increasing carbs in the diet was also promoted at one time even by the government. Although food choices have gone through several changes, frequent eating has become a habit. The food is spread all around us. You can get hundreds of fast food joints on your way that are selling food items that are tempting and cheap. It may not cost you much time and money to grab a bite on your way. However, this habit of munching all the time is taking us towards the health doom. This habit would have to be changed.

Most people are scared of the thought that they may not be able to eat what they want. In intermittent fasting, it doesn't work like that. You will still be free to eat practically everything in a limit so that temptation for food can be avoided. However, you will have to follow some reasonable restraint. The habit of eating 'ad libitum' or whenever you desire will have to be controlled. This is very easy when you make some positive changes in your food choices. In any case, there will not be severe restraints in your eating windows. There is no reason to worry as you will be free to eat the things you want in this period. The major portion of the fasting window passes in your sleep, and hence, the chances of temptation are very few and far between. You can expect an easy ride in this section as long as you are ready to curb your habit of frequent snacking.

- **Food Choices**

Most people feel that they'd never be able to get any success through diets as avoiding certain foods is not possible for them. There is no doubt in the fact that food has a strong impact on the physique. We are what we eat. The kind of food we eat eventually becomes a part of our body. Therefore, if you are eating a lot of trashy food, it can never have a healthy impact on you. However, it is also correct that your body has a very robust system of discarding the bad and keeping the good, and hence, there is a tolerance limit even for bad foods.

So, you can get in shape even if you are taking some liberties in food. However, this should always remain in a limit, and you should always try to eliminate such things from your food slowly.

Refined sugar, alcohol, fried food, highly processed food items, or foods that are made from refined flours are examples of what can hurt your health. You must always try to avoid these items. If that is not entirely possible, you should at least try to limit your intake of foods high in sugars, refined flours, and more.

Intermittent fasting is not a routine that limits your life. It means that once in a while, you can have cheat days and cheat meals where you can eat some of the foods that may be discouraged on this eating plan. You don't have to feel cut-off from your friends and social circle because you can't eat certain things. However, you shouldn't make it a habit or a regular occurrence; responsible eating will not hurt your health goals.

- **Healthy Routine and Exercise**

Exercise is very important for a healthy body either you are following intermittent fasting or not. Therefore, it is not a contentious subject. Exercise will accelerate weight loss and will also help you in getting healthier. Moderate exercise is good for the functioning of your heart and improving your immune system. Intense physical activity is important if you want to lose a lot of weight fast. It also helps in muscle building.

Exercise helps your weight loss and health goals. However, while fasting, certain things need to be kept in mind. Women shouldn't do high-intensity exercises on the fasting days and must keep one-day intervals to give the body complete rest. Exercising in the fasting state is especially very helpful if you are trying to burn fat as the HGH and adrenaline hormone levels are very high in that state. They not only help in burning the fat considerably faster, but they also increase your stamina and boost muscle growth. Detailed tips on exercise and the ones that are especially helpful will be given in the exercise section.

Therefore, including exercise in your daily routine is always very helpful. The kind of exercise you want to do would depend upon your weight loss goal. However, including at least brisk exercises in the schedule is very important for good health. So, you would be required to make certain changes in your lifestyle in all three areas if you want to get the best results from intermittent fasting.

As a fast recap:

1. You would need to make changes in your eating patterns. You will have to follow strict eating and fasting windows. You will also have to reduce the number of meals consumed in a day.

2. Including healthy food items in your meals is always very helpful. You will be able to remain much healthier, and your weight would also go fast if you stop consuming fast food, processed items, fried food, and other such things. However, you can eat practically most of the things once in a while responsibly.

3. Exercise is important for keeping the body healthy, and it also helps in your weight loss journey. Dedicating some time to exercise every day would be very helpful.

Food - The Changes You Need to Make

One fact that has been repeated several times is that what you eat and how much you eat doesn't play a very significant role in intermittent fasting. This may look like a very incredulous claim.

Although it is true, yet you would have to take it with a pinch of salt.

- **You Can Eat Practically Everything But With Restraint**

Eating almost everything and still lose weight comes with a condition. The condition is that you can only eat that thing once in a while and that too in reasonable quantities. It means that if your mind is craving to have desserts that you know isn't good, and then you will have only two choices.

First, you can suppress the desire and keep sulking. The result of such suppressions generally is a weakened resolve to continue the practice. The temptation keeps building, and soon you'd reach the threshold where it would be difficult to control anymore. Most people don't continue their weight loss measures after some breaches as they feel that they are not cut out of it and compromise with their weight. Second, you can choose to eat it once in a while or on designated cheat days and never let the temptation build inside you. This way you'd never feel like a total failure. Every cheat day would feel liberating and wouldn't fill you with guilt. It would be easier for you to continue.

However, the main purpose of this freedom is to keep you on track, but it shouldn't be taken for granted. I believe that after you have been following intermittent fasting, you learn to cope with such temptations and the need for cheat days vanishes.

Therefore, we understand that once in a while, you can eat anything. You must try to avoid certain things like fast food, fried things, sweets, sweet chocolates, carbonated drinks, alcohol, and processed items as they are addictive and unhealthy. They would lead to cravings and make fasting difficult for you.

- **You Do Not Need to Count Calories**

One of the biggest problems with many people is that they start feeling disheartened simply from the fact that they would have to cut calories. The best thing about intermittent fasting is that you do not need to cut calories at all. You don't even need to count calories to see if you are consuming more or fewer calories. You must eat the amount of food that makes you satisfied. As long as you are eating healthy things, excess calories don't matter much in intermittent fasting.

It is essential that your meals have all the macro-ingredients in the required proportions. If you are focused on losing fat; then your meals must have high-fat, low-carb, and medium protein diet. You don't need to worry from the fact that for reducing fat you are being advised to eat fat as we will be explaining that fact.

Fat, protein, and carbohydrates play a very crucial role in your health. If you are not eating them in good proportion, you will always feel energy drained. Therefore, it is important that your meals have a good mix of the three.

Ideally, the proportion of these macronutrients should be:

Fat: 65-70% - You should take your fats from healthy things like eggs, chicken, fish, avocado, nuts, beef, olive oil, and other solid fats. You must try to buy as much fresh and healthy food as possible. Try to avoid canned or preserved items as the chemicals affect your body too.

Fat has almost double the calories in the same amount of food when compared to carbs. That means that even if you are eating food in small quantity, you will be getting the required amount of fat. The fat is very satisfying, and it also helps you in going from one meal to another without feeling the urge to have snacks. So, fat should be the main part of your meals. Increasing the quantity of fat in the meals would help you in kick-starting the ketosis process.

Proteins: 20-25% - Proteins are required for building muscles and tissues and other structural things in the body. Your body cannot produce protein on its own, and hence, protein must be a part of your meals. 20-25% of the calories should come from your protein intake. Remember, if you reduce the quantity of protein consumed, your body may face problems in building muscles, and you may also face the loss of muscle mass.

Good sources of protein are eggs, chicken, lean meats, fish, beans, legumes, etc. Try to eat as much organic food as possible. Although protein is essential for your body, you must not overdo protein intake. It means if you are consuming protein in high quantity, then it will not help your cause of weight loss much as your liver will convert the excess protein into glucose. Production of glucose is one thing that needs to be discouraged as you want to start ketosis for weight loss.

Carbs: 5-10% - Carbohydrates have never been our primary food source. Our ancestors didn't know the art of cultivation, and that situation prevailed for thousands of years. This means that during this time, their main source of food was animal meat. The only source of carbohydrate was fruits that they gathered. Fruits are full of micronutrients, vitamins, and minerals. They are also rich in dietary fiber. Hence, eating fruit is healthy as they give your gut the fiber to help the digestion process and also provide the micronutrients.

However, these days, carbs are our main source of fuel. We are living a carb dependent life. Bread, cakes, chips, fries, crackers, buns, and other such things are made of refined flour and sugar. The digestion time for these things is very short, and they instantly spike our blood sugar levels. But, the energy provided by these things is short-lived, and you start feeling the need to eat again very soon. Carbs also leave a lot of waste during glucose conversion. These are the things that you would need to avoid as much as possible.

The carbs should give more than 5-10% of the calories in your meals. You should only include healthy carbs like whole grains, non-starchy green leafy vegetables, and fruits for carbs. These things are full of fiber that slows down your digestive process, and you keep feeling fuller even hours after consuming your last meal. This solves the problem of cravings and hunger pangs. The fiber is also very important for improving your digestive tract issues and also helps in reducing inflammation. It cleans your intestines and your colon. Some health issues can be solved by increasing fiber in your diet.

You must give special emphasis to non-starchy green leafy vegetables in your diet. Spinach, kale, and other such vegetables have a lot of soluble fiber, vitamins, and minerals. They would help you a lot in staying healthy. They are also full of antioxidants that help in fighting chronic inflammation. You wouldn't have to worry about counting the number of calories while consuming green leafy vegetables, as they only add a negligible amount of calories and you must not count them.

All these things have to be consumed in a rough estimate, as the things that provide you protein also provide fat. Even if you consume a bit more in your meals, you don't have to worry, as your body will balance everything. In intermittent fasting, calories matter less and the number of times you eat and the time you eat matters more.

Chapter 10 - Intermittent Fasting and the Process of Autophagy

The reason why many of us go through a detox diet or even juice cleanses is that we want to get rid of the toxins in our body. The thing is about juice cleanses and detox diets is that it does not flush toxins out of your body as fast as you expect, although there is nothing wrong with having a juice cleanse.

Do you want to flush out toxins from your body? If that is what you want to do, there is another way to optimize the way our body cleanses itself from toxins and this is the process of autophagy.

What is Autophagy?

Autophagy is one of the most powerful cleaning processes carried out by the body. Recently, a Japanese scientist Dr. Yoshinori Oshumi won the Nobel peace prize in 2016 for his research on the concept. He found that the body had a unique ability to purge all the bad elements in the body including the malformed proteins, pathogens, unwanted infections that are harming the body if it senses an acute shortage of energy. This means that if a person is starving, the body would turn off all the bad process in the body and would start using them to produce energy. It would become a highly efficient machine to survive for the longest.

This process can also be used for great advantage as it gives the unique opportunity to get rid of most of the diseases. Even the progression of scariest diseases like cancer can be slowed down with by inducing autophagy. To initiate autophagy, you do not need to do anything extra. You need to stop adding these extras to your body, and the process would begin on its own.

What triggers autophagy?

Fasting is the only way through which autophagy can begin. Studies have further shown that although long fasts are more effective in initiating autophagy, it can also begin with fasts as small as 12-14 hours every day. This means that by following intermittent fasting, you can get the unique advantages of autophagy. Autophagy is the ultimate solution for most of the diseases in the body. It can treat diseases and bring longevity. You would feel younger and healthier if your body is going through autophagy. It is a process in which your body is utilizing all the waste products to produce energy and cells. Nothing gets wasted, and every resource is put to best use.

The purpose of this chapter is to tell you how intermittent fasting can help you in getting holistic health. It is not some fad diet that merely helps in losing weight which is only a temporary resort and not even a solution. If your overall health is good, weight management will become effortless, and this is the main aim of intermittent fasting.

Intermittent fasting opens the doors of holistic health for you. It makes staying healthy and fit very easy without having to go through the torturous routine of elaborate diets that don't even give you enough to eat. You wouldn't have to keep feeling restricted and desperate through the whole process as eating some of the things becomes a dream. Intermittent fasting will give you great freedom and ease of life. You will have to follow some basic rules, and the doors of good health will open for you without having to spend large sums of money or time.

Sounds good. So how does autophagy benefit me?

Autophagy plays a huge role in controlling inflammation as well as boosting immunity. Apart from boosting immunity, autophagy has been found to benefit the body in these forms:

- Preventing cancer
- Neurodegenerative disorders
- Inflammatory diseases

- Infections
- Lessing aging symptoms
- Insulin resistance

Also, studies point out that the lack of autophagy in the body could also be harmful since the body is not given enough time to get rid of toxins and this leads to higher cholesterol, lethargy, weight gain as well as impaired brain function. Autophagy makes our body more efficient and it stops cancerous growths as well as metabolic dysfunction such as diabetes and obesity.

Autophagy and Anti-Aging

In the science of aging, autophagy is a crucial breakthrough and while this has been known to scientists way back in the 1950s, the past decade or so has there been an intense conversation around autophagy and its effects on improving our overall cellular health. Research published in the Journal of Clinical Experimental Pathology mentions that autophagy has the ability to remove accumulated toxic deposits to promote cell rejuvenation and maintenance by using recycled components as an alternative nutrient reserve.

The research also suggests that autophagy promotes longevity because it enables organisms to recover much rapidly when there is stress-induced damage on a cellular level. This research says that cells have the ability to effectively clean and remove the damage which allows them to function better. In more layman terms, autophagy allows the body's cells to more efficiently.

Holistic Benefits of Autophagy

- **It enhances our body's metabolic capacity -** Autophagy can be activated to improve the body's mitochondria at its deepest cellular level. This makes the cells work better and eventually makes cells becomes resilient.

- **It prevents or lessens neurodegenerative disorders -** Many of these disorders happen due to damaged protein cells that form around and in neurons. The process of autophagy protects the body and its cells from preventing neurodegenerative issues from taking place such as those associated with Parkinson's Huntington's diseases as well as Alzheimer's.

- **It helps fight against infectious diseases -** autophagy removes toxins that create infections and it also removes how the immune system of the body responds to infections.

- **It improves your muscle performance** - When we exercise, we focus stress on our cells and this makes energy go up and some of your body parts get worn out faster. Through the process of autophagy, it will eliminate some of this damage and maintain a healthy energy level check.

- **It prevents cancer growth** - if none of the benefits above you are attractive enough, then this might want you to fast so you can trigger autophagy. Autophagy suppresses the processes related to cancer development. These processes are such as damaged DNA as well as chronic inflammation of organs.

The research and study done on autophagy tell us that this process makes our body perform better because it clears out cellular junk and it gives way for cells to build themselves with better parts. It is a biological upgrade.

How can you activate Autophagy?

We know that fasting is the only way to activate autophagy. But let's take a deeper look into how this happens. Autography is triggered when our body is on a stress-response mode. When we stress our cells through fasting, it is a natural way to stress the body and turn on the process of autophagy.

Intermittent fasting is an excellent way to activate autophagy because it creates nutrient deprivation in your cells. Exercise is another way to create cellular stress. Any kind of fasting period for more than 16 hours is an excellent period to trigger autophagy.

Chapter 11 - Myths Concerning Intermittent Fasting

As much as we like to admit it, when we embark on a new diet plan or a new eating system or anything to do with food and weight loss, we want to know if it works. We also want to know if the effort we are putting in will actually see results and also how fast will you see results.

It's normal to have questions and concerns, which is why we read up on what the plan we want to follow, we do a little research on the internet to see what the experts say, we read books like this to give us information on how to do it, what are the best practices, and how to make it to work for you. While the primary information in this book is to provide you with guidance, this chapter specifically aims to dispel myths or misconceptions concerning intermittent fasting.

Many people do not fully understand intermittent fasting, and they are going to start talking about it with a lot of misconceptions and other issues as well. But despite all of these, intermittent fasting is an effective way to improve your health and help you to start feeling amazing in no time.

Add on the great weight loss benefits, and it won't be long before you start using fasting as your go-to tool for better health. However, we are going to spend a bit of time in this chapter taking a look at some of the common misconceptions that often show up in regards to intermittent fasting so you know the truth and the lies about this great eating plan.

- **You could ruin your health**

Intermittent fasting is one of the best ways to stay healthy. It will improve your overall health biomarkers and will keep you healthy. There are so many health benefits that come from intermittent fasting from reducing your heart health risks to losing weight, preventing diabetes, and even making your life easier so you feel less stress!

- **You could end up starving!**

Starvation mode is bad as far as fat burning is concerned, and there is no doubt about it. If your body goes into starvation mode, then it will lower the metabolic functions to a bare minimum. You would feel energy drained and would become lethargic. However, intermittent fasting can never lead to starvation mode.

It would take anywhere between 72-96 hours for the starvation mode to kick in. It means that simply by fasting for 24 hours or less, you can never enter starvation mode. Although there is a lot of paranoia about the starvation mode, it is a healthy state in which your body starts serious restructuring, and many serious diseases can get cured on their own by an internal process called autophagy in this mode. There is no reason for you to fear the starvation mode and you can never enter starvation mode simply by following intermittent fasting. You will have to follow much longer fasts for that.

- **You could lose all that hard-earned muscle mass**

It is a popular misconception that once your blood sugar levels go down the body would basically start with cannibalism and eat away its muscles. It doesn't work that way. Our bodies have passed through millions of years of evolution and nature had better plans. It is true that when the readily available glucose ends, the glycogen stores are burned, and then the body starts consuming the extra amino acids. However, these amino acids are those that cannot be converted into muscles. It is protein but not the one that can be utilized. If not consumed by the body, this protein would get excreted from your body the next day.

So, there is no reason to worry about losing muscle mass. The body wouldn't start eating its own muscles; it would begin ketosis once readily available energy gets exhausted, and fat burning then begins. Protein releases a very small amount of energy, and the conversion takes a lot of effort. It isn't an efficient process for your body, at least not as efficient as metabolizing fat or glucose. Loss of muscle mass would only start after very long periods of starvation when there is no more fat left for the body to burn. It only shows up when you have been starving yourself for a long time, and there isn't any fat or glucose left for the body to go through.

- **You could trigger more stress responses than you already have**

People believe that fasting would lead to a stress response in the body, and they would be correct. Intermittent fasting does invoke a little amount of stress. However, this is a good type of stress that helps your body. In fact, you are barely going to notice this stress, but it will do wonders with helping you to handle some of the bigger stressors in your life.

- **You need 6 meals a day for a faster metabolism**

This is a myth that has led to the highest amount of damage to public health in general. Only a small amount of energy is used to convert food into energy. So, if you feel that by eating a higher number of meals in a day you would be spending more calories, you are wrong. A higher number of meals would ultimately lead to the consumption of a greater number of calories, and it also leads to insulin resistance and other such health issues.

Bottom Line

Celebrities such as Terry Crews, Miranda Kerr, Hugh Jackman as well as Ben Affleck are all followers of the 16-hour fast. If you are unable to eliminate a food group (such as carbs in a Keto diet), then Intermittent Fasting is a safe and healthy route to go with if weight loss, insulin regulation, and anti-aging goals are what you are looking for.

Chapter bonus - The Four Pillars of Successful Intermittent Fasting

Intermittent fasting is a lifestyle choice. It isn't just a fad diet that you pick and let go off when you reach a goal. By this chapter, you would already have read the amazing benefits of intermittent fasting that has more to do then just fat loss and because of this, you can incorporate intermittent fasting as a healthy lifestyle routine rather than a diet. When doing intermittent fasting as a lifestyle, remember that is not about filling your body with empty calories or even putting your body through psychological and physiological stress. You want to intermittent fast the right way and the healthy way.

What are the right and healthy way?

1 - Firstly, start with choosing a method that works for you. The easiest is the 16/:8 method followed by the 5:2 method. Do what works best for your lifestyle as well as your climate, surroundings, and access to wholesome food.

2 - Stick to one method at a time. If you have chosen the Warrior method, stick to it. Or if you stick to a 16/8 method, stick to it. Do not go back and forth between methods because this will mess up with your digestive system and your hormones.

3 - Create a routine. Routine makes it easier for you to identify what hours work best for you to manage the things in your life. While not everything is within your control, establishing certain rules help you stick to your plan. For example, if breakfast is something you need to have, then create a routine around it with your intermittent fasting.

4 - Never overdo it. If for some reason you are hungry or you feel nauseous or you are sick or you've done too much of physical work that you are hungry and fatigued, do not force the fast. Eat if you need to.

5 - Eat healthy. There is no point going through an eating plan or diet or fast if what you're putting into your mouth is processed foods. Intermittent fasts, keto diets, etc only work well if you focus on eating wholesome foods, unprocessed meats, and grains and drinking plenty of water.

Now that you've established some rules, here is four-pillar guidance to help you focus on making the intermittent fast work for you in the long run.

To do this, you need to focus on:

1. Setting your Goals
2. Creating the right environment
3. Exercise
4. Sticking to a routine

Let's have a look at how all of these four aspects are the pillars of a successful intermittent fasting lifestyle.

1. Setting the Goals for your Fast

What do you want to achieve with intermittent fasting? Weight loss? Insulin regulation? Better weight management?

Setting correct goals is very important if you want to succeed in anything. Right goals keep you motivated on the way and help you in moving ahead. If you set wrong or impossible goals, then there is a high probability that you'll start getting demotivated very early in the process.

Fighting obesity is a tough goal. Millions of people in the US alone are fighting with this menace and most of them surrender at one point of the other. It isn't the sheer failure of the procedure that leads to giving up. Their unreal expectations, unrealistic goals, and ambiguous milestones lead to disappointment.

There is a simple thing, if you are working towards something, then the results can be slow, but they'll be there. It is a simple matter of cause and effect. Every action reacts. However, if you are not witnessing any result, then it can mean that you are making some horrible mistake somewhere and to judge that too you would have to set milestones. Therefore, setting clear, realistic, and achievable goals is very important.

Intermittent fasting is a long-term solution, and it brings a substantial change in your life. Although you may see swift changes in your weight, other health effects take time in surfacing as body corrects the processes slowly and naturally. So, your goal setting would depend upon the kind of result you are looking for. If you are going to follow intermittent fasting for overcoming problems like insulin resistance, diabetes, and chronic inflammation, then your goals need to be long-term. You cannot expect any visible change in the short-term.

Set Small but Clear Milestones

Setting milestones is very important if you are chasing a big target to keep ensuring that you are moving in the right direction and keep checking that your efforts are bringing results. You can't keep chasing a target for a year and then realize that the efforts have been in vain. That would be painful, disappointing, and disheartening.

For weight loss and burning the belly fat, you must set short-term goals. You must set goals like you would lose certain pounds in a month. You must not get greedy while setting goals and always set goals that can be realized. Try to make changes in your goals if you have not been able to realize the goals in the previous months. Consistently failing to achieve goals will bring down your morale.

It is also important to remember that weighing scale may not be the right way to measure your progress while following intermittent fasting. You would initially lose weight, but later on, the weight loss may stop, but you will still be burning fat, and hence, you must always use both the parameters.

If you are not able to achieve your monthly goals in any specific month, you must not get worried as that can happen due to some reasons and it may only be a one-off incident. Getting in panic mode wouldn't be very helpful. You must view your progress on average.

Set Long Term Goals

Intermittent fasting aims to help you in improving the overall health biomarkers. Over some time, you'd not only start feeling light but more energetic and healthier. Your immunity would increase, and you would also be able to feel better internally.

However, these are the things that can't be measured without technical help. If you want to measure this, you must take a through a blood test and look for the things that haven't been working correctly. Checking the mean blood sugar levels, lipid profile for measuring cholesterol, liver, and kidney function tests, etc. can give you a clear picture of your health. These tests would help you better in assessing the changes in your health when you measure the same after a year or so. Whatever be your goal, it should be clear, and you must work towards it in a focused way. It helps a lot in remaining sincere in the efforts.

2. Creating the Right Environment

Success in any aspect of life never happens in a total vacuum. An individuals' determination, will power, intelligence, and a little bit of luck determine the outcome of success. Apart from variables that you can control, there is also the surrounding environment that you are in and the outside circumstances that often influence success rates.

In order to achieve the goals you have set when you go through intermittent fasting, you need to pay attention and take control of whichever type of environments that you surround yourself with on a regular basis. No matter how strong or smart you are, if you are in the wrong group or environment - it will be very difficult for you to achieve your goals. Why? Because your external environment has some degree of influence on the state of your mind – the way you think, what is right, what's wrong, and also the way you behave. Your thoughts and behavior will be especially influenced by the people you surround yourself on a daily basis and also the kinds of places you spend most of your time in.

Birds of a Feather

Hans. F Hansen, the former Scandinavian football player, said 'People inspire you, or they drain you, pick wisely'. His words cannot ring truer than this. The first portion of our environment that influences our success has got to be the people we deal with daily. In 2013, research published in an issue of Psychological Science found that if you surround yourself with friends who were determined and driven to achieve the same goals as you, you become determined and driven too.

The same is said if you were a negative environment. If you surround yourself with friends who lead an unhealthy way of life, the chances of you becoming unhealthy and gain weight yourself are very likely. Similarly, if you hang with people who always eat fast food, then you'd end up eating fast food all the time too.

More and more research is being conducted to understand human interactions, especially those related to the types of people who become part of our social circle. Our social circle affects almost every, if not all, aspects of our lives - from work to relationships, to business, to life at home, school, and even at a party. So when you list out your personal goals, commitments, and personal statement, think about the people currently in your circle - are any of them holding you back?

All of us have choices. So instead of surrounding yourself with negativity and spending time with people who make you hate life or hate the way you look, who make you give up easily, spend time with people who make you appreciate and love life! Spend time with those that motivate you and help you become a better person and one that can stick to your intermittent fasting goals. Being in a healthy relationship is one of the most important characteristics of being a successful person. Having the right people in your life will give you that extra boost when obstacles come your way. They will be your anchor, your support and your motivation to move on.

Altering the Environment you are in

Apart from hanging out with people who can help you stay focused on your goals, the second feature in our environment that influences our success rate is the places we spend our time at. An environment that increases productivity and allows freedom of expression is a great place to spend your time in as it will motivate and inspire you. Apart from choosing your friends, you must also take ownership of where you spend most of your time in. A conducive environment keeps your positive juices flowing, stimulates the senses, and gives you less distraction. You can do various little changes to alter your space whether at home or in the office.

Here are a few things you can do to switch up your environment to ensure you stick to your fasting goals:

• Creating a clutter-free space

The way we keep our home and office spaces is a valuable way of ensuring that our goals are met. Imagine coming home to a living room with so much clutter, it makes it hard for you to exercise or even meditate. Or what if your entire pantry and fridge are filled with tins and cans and boxes of food you don't even know are edible or not which makes it hard for you to even meal plan. Decluttering your house, office, and of course, fridge and pantry help you know what goes where, what you have to cook a meal, reduces stress as well as time to look for things and overall gives you a clear mind to focus on your goals.

• Adding a little bit of positivity wherever you go

Simple things can truly make a difference in our mindset. Sometimes, we need a little pick-me-up to maintain a clear head. For instance, placing a mini potted plant or a mini fountain on your office desk can dramatically alter the presence of your workspace. Similarly, instead of running on the treadmill every time you hit the gym, change it to doing a few laps outside the gym - somewhere where you can breathe in the fresh air, get a little sun, step out into the outdoors - then come inside the gym and continue your strength workouts.

Countless studies done have shown the impact of nature in our lives - just by surrounding ourselves with nature can dramatically improve our focus, minimize stress, and increase cognitive ability. Live in an apartment? Then create a balcony garden! String up fairy lights, put in a few potted plants, and you can great a tiny oasis right in the comfort of your own home.

Apart from plants and mini fountains, you can also paste up motivational quotes and sayings that have an impact on the goal you want to achieve. It is always great to have your own personal motivation mantra. Find a quote you like, get it printed out in whatever color you want, and stick it right next to the goals that you have written down. You can also create a vision board - get images that are visually appealing and related to your goals. Go bold with the designs and colors so your mind is easily attracted to it and it will instantly make you feel good and set your mind and energy right.

- Creating a workspace that motivates

The office space is the longest time most of us spend our daily life and it is also the place where you can express your freedom easily. So even though your office space is hell in fluorescent lighting, create an oasis that works for you- something that reflects your personal interests and your values, something that inspires and motivates you. Your mind is the only one holding you from breaking your fast and sitting the entire day in your office desk can make us bored and want to munch. Your workspace may be the last thing you think about when you are on a fast, you work here every day so it will influence some amount of your success and inspiration, whether you are aware of it or not. This relates to your fitness goals and your fasting goals. Keeping an organized and motivating workspace will guarantee positive outcomes.

At the end of the day, an environment that brings out the best in you is essential. Part of ensuring that you stick to your intermittent fast is about being aware of the people you surround yourself with and the places that you interact with. Think about how you can make changes to these spaces so that it serves you better. If these people and spaces do not benefit you in any way and only bring you down, then get rid of it or spend less time in it. Life is too short to mix with people who are only out to make your life worse and bring you down.

3. Exercise

Exercise is an important element in maintaining a healthy body and mind. Many people resort to diets and fasts and cleanse simply because they want a quick and easy way out to lose weight.

The secret to maintaining a healthy and balanced weight is to maintain a calorie balance by eating the right foods as well as to optimize the body's natural way of releasing toxins. Exercise is an excellent way the body can burn fats as well as release toxins and together with intermittent fasting, you have a sustainable and healthy journey towards maintaining your ideal weight.

Picking the Right Kind of Exercise

Picking out the right exercises to go with intermittent fasting can give your weight loss goals a considerable boost when you are nearing the completion of your 14-16 hour fast, the strength peaks. This is the time to give your body the biggest push. You would be able to work out hard and get the most out of it.

There are two highly supporting hormones during this period. HGH and Adrenaline production is very high by the end of the fasting period. These hormones help in increasing your strength and stamina; they also accelerate the fat burning and muscle building. You should exercise on an empty stomach, and generally, all kinds of workouts can be done by men. Cardio, weightlifting, strength training, and HIIT would bring great results. However, women should limit themselves to cardio, aerobics, light exercises, or yoga on fasting days.

The kind of exercise you can do would also depend upon the type of food you are having. If you are still having carb-rich meals, then you may feel depleted in the morning as carbs do not provide energy for long. If you want to do high-intensity exercise, then you should start taking a nutrient-dense diet which has the macros balanced. If you are having apprehensions about your ability to work out hard after a full night of fasting, your fears are baseless. Muscles have their glycogen stores, and you wouldn't feel a problem in exercising.

For Better Results You can Do the Following:

Match Your Meals with Your Routine

Your meals have an impact on your performance and endurance. Therefore, you must select your meal wisely. If you are trying to bulk muscles and would be doing weight lifting, then the percentage of protein should be higher in your meals.

If you are trying to burn fat, then you should increase the amount of fat in your diet because increasing fat in the diet would lead to fat loss eventually. If you are trying to detox your body and would only be doing cardio or yoga, you can have a normal diet with the right mix of essential nutrients.

Always Remain Hydrated

Remaining hydrated is very important. Drink a lot of water, and especially during exercise and after it, drink a lot of electrolytes as there would be a loss of minerals and your body would need electrolytes for replenishing its stores.

Don't Push Yourself Too Hard

HIIT or high-intensity interval training is the best during intermittent fasting as it prevents excessive muscle damage and helps in building them. Doing the same exercise for too long can have adverse effects.

4. Sticking to a Routine

In decluttering our spaces, we also need to think about decluttering our routine. One of the implicit benefits of intermittent fasting is that it makes meals simpler and it also makes your routine simpler. When we fast intermittently, we are already confining our eating periods to a specific time frame. This is already a routine but to ensure that you stick to this eating time frame, you need to relook the other aspects of your daily life and ensure that it positively contributes to your feasting and fasting times.

One way to do this is by creating a morning and bedtime routine.

First Lady Michelle Obama's morning routine is described as such in her interview for O, The Oprah Magazine in 2009. "If I had to get up to take care of my kids, I'd get up to do that. But when it comes to yourself, then it's suddenly, 'Oh, I can't get up at 4:30.' So I had to change that. If I don't exercise, I won't feel good. I'll get depressed." Anna Wintour, Vogue Editor-in-Chief starts her day at 5.45 AM with a vigorous tennis match. AOL CEO, Tim Armstrong gets out of bed at 5 or 5.15 AM to answer emails or sneak in a workout. As mentioned in previous chapters, starting small is always a good thing. So, here's an example of a morning routine you can start off with:

- Start by waking up at least one hour earlier than your usual time.
- Make your bed. Military training always places the importance of soldiers making their bed perfectly. The reason is simply that you've accomplished one task in the morning!
- Drink a glass of lemon water. Lemon water in the morning is known to boost energy and brainpower. A few slices of lemon, cucumber, or mint leaves in your morning water will not break your fast.
- Do some light stretching to get your blood pumping and awaken your senses.
- Listen to your favorite songs during the shower. Songs give you a better mood to kick off the day!

Since we have done a morning routine when you wake up, creating a morning routine at work is also essential to get yourself organized to be productive. Having all these different routines helps make your self-disciplined. A great app to use would be Coach.me and this can help you maintain and stick to your good habits. While at work, look around your workspace- is it in good order? Do you have things organized?

Next, look at the people you speak with or have lunch with. How long do your meetings take? What kind of person is your boss? When you get back home, reflect on all these items. See how you can improve your social circle and work environment by doing little changes along the way. Write down the actions that you want to take the next day.

For example, if you have a fitness goal but you have a very desk-based job that does not allow you to move so much, maybe for the next few days, walk to lunch? Or do little exercises while at the desk? For those who have a career based goal, maybe you want to look at what you do the first thing in the morning. Do you spend so much time procrastinating by going through social media and Facebook? Think about the things that you want to do the first thing you get into your office. Here's an example of how your morning routine at work can be:

- Switch on your computer. Make a cup of coffee.
- Read the newspaper.
- Speak to your co-workers can catch up on work-related business.

- Check your calendar to see what you have scheduled the whole week.
- Do tasks that require your immediate attention.
- Reply to emails.

Night Routine

Bedtime is more of a time to reflect. It is a time for you to calm your senses and switch off from the world.

1. Start by switching off. Research shows that you should stop looking at your digital devices 15 minutes before you go to sleep.
2. Do some light stretching to relax and soothe yourself.
3. Say a prayer, do some reflection or just meditate in savasana.
4. Kiss your partner/spouse and children goodnight.
5. Breathe deeply, through a long inhale and a slow exhale while keeping your eyes closed. This will enable you to fall into a deep sleep, faster.

Bottom Line

By creating the right environment we are much more equipped to fulfill our goals compared to having an environment that works against our journey towards success. As mentioned earlier, intermittent fasting is more about a lifestyle change rather than a one-off diet fad.

When you start intermittent fasting, you simplify meals times and this affects your daily routine, making it simpler to follow through. Simplifying the processes, your actions, and the number of ways to get things done will ultimately make it easier to follow through with intermittent fasting making it sustainable and healthy.

Conclusion

You've made it through this book! Congratulations.

How do you feel? At which point did you begin your intermittent fasting when you first opened the pages of this book?

Whatever point you decided to start with your intermittent fast, the point is that you started a journey towards better health both internally and externally. Most people begin intermittent fasting because their ultimate goal is to lose weight but after reading all the other benefits and also experiencing these benefits yourself, intermittent fasting might come to something that you would do regularly and that's the great thing about this eating plan - it can be done on a long term basis compared to other eating plans such as the keto diet for example.

You have all the information about intermittent fasting that you need, and hopefully, it will help you make the best out of your journey towards becoming a better, healthier, and happier version of yourself.

You must always remember that this eating plan needs to be followed properly but please take note that while it may be beneficial, it may not necessarily be suitable for everyone because not everybody is going to have the same body type or health level.

Speaking to your doctor before you began will help you identify if this eating plan is medically suitable for you. Sometimes, we feel like we are not losing weight or hitting your body goals not because we are eating too much or not exercising enough. It is probably because of hormones and speaking to your doctor will help confirm this.

Intermittent fasting, at the end of the day, is a method that is supposed to help you better your health, so please remember to always listen to your body at every step of the way, especially during your workout sessions. Never push your body beyond more than what it is supposed to be doing, because the last thing you want is to set yourself back by getting injured or worse.

If intermittent fasting is a journey that is not just about weight loss, but about better health for you, remember that the road to losing weight and keeping it off is a long-term one, and there is no solution that is going to provide you with overnight results (if only that were possible!). Always put your health, safety, and wellbeing above all else, even weight loss and consult your doctor if at any point you feel uncomfortable along the way.

Good luck!

Finally, if you found this book useful in any way, a review on Amazon is always appreciated!

www.ingramcontent.com/pod-product-compliance
Lightning Source LLC
Chambersburg PA
CBHW061810250726
48657CB00001B/369